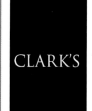

CLARK'S

ESSENTIAL
GUIDE TO

MAMMOGRAPHY

CLARK'S COMPANION ESSENTIAL GUIDES

Series Editor
A. Stewart Whitley

Clark's Essential Guide to Clinical Ultrasound
Jan Dodgeon and Gill Harrison

Clark's Essential Guide to Mammography
Claire Borrelli and Claire Mercer

Clark's Essential PACS, RIS and Imaging Informatics
Alexander Peck

Clark's Essential Physics in Imaging for Radiographers, Second Edition
Ken Holmes, Marcus Elkington and Phil Harris

https://www.routledge.com/Clarks-Companion-Essential-Guides/book-series/CRCCLACOMESS

Also available in the Clark's Family:

Clark's Positioning in Radiography, Thirteenth Edition
A. Stewart Whitley, Gail Jefferson, Ken Holmes, Graham Hoadley, Charles Sloane and Craig Anderson

Clark's Pocket Handbook for Radiographers, Second Edition
A. Stewart Whitley, Charles Sloane, Gail Jefferson, Ken Holmes and Craig Anderson

**Clark's Procedures in Diagnostic Imaging:
A System-Based Approach**
A. Stewart Whitley, Jan Dodgeon, Angela Meadows, Jane Cullingworth, Ken Holmes, Marcus Jackson, Graham Hoadley and Randeep Kulshrestha

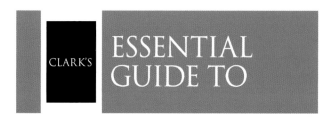

MAMMOGRAPHY

Claire Borrelli
Head of Education & Clinical Training
St George's National Breast Education Centre, London, UK
Radiographic Advisor to the NHSBSP/NHSE, UK

Claire Mercer
Head of Radiography
School of Health and Society
University of Salford, Salford, UK

Series Editor for *Clark's Companion Essential Guides:*

A. Stewart Whitley
Former ISRRT Director of Professional Practice &
Radiology Advisor, UK Radiology Advisory Services
Preston, Lancashire, UK

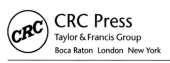

CRC Press
Taylor & Francis Group
Boca Raton London New York

CRC Press is an imprint of the
Taylor & Francis Group, an **informa** business

First edition published 2024
by CRC Press
6000 Broken Sound Parkway NW, Suite 300, Boca Raton, FL 33487-2742

and by CRC Press
4 Park Square, Milton Park, Abingdon, Oxon, OX14 4RN

CRC Press is an imprint of Taylor & Francis Group, LLC

ISBN: 9781032033655 (hbk)
ISBN: 9781032033624 (pbk)
ISBN: 9781003186939 (ebk)

DOI: 10.1201/9781003186939

Typeset in Linotype Berling LT Std
by Evolution Design & Digital

CONTENTS

Contents

FOREWORD

It has been a delight to witness the development and publication of *Clark's Essential Guide to Mammography*. This latest addition to the *Clark's* series of pocket and desktop books is a testament to the skills, knowledge, and dedication of the authors, who are key members of the radiography profession and who have at heart the desire to share their knowledge and experience with radiographers and image practitioners engaged in mammography in the many and varied diagnostic image settings.

Miss K. C. Clark, I am sure, would welcome this important addition to the series, which has its origins in the recently published *Clark's Procedures in Diagnostic Imaging (A System-Based Approach)* which included a 'Breast Imaging' chapter dedicated to the detection of breast pathology.

This book, however, is dedicated specifically to the use of mammography and will be a valuable aid and resource for the those engaged in the breast care and healthcare communities.

This book conveys to its readers an immense amount of important knowledge that is current and relevant and essential to modern-day mammography practice.

The service users must surely benefit by this publication.

A. Stewart Whitley
Series Editor
Former ISRRT Director of Professional Practice &
Radiology Advisor
UK Radiology Advisory Services
Preston, Lancashire, UK

PREFACE

Clark's Essential Guide to Mammography is part of the *Clark's* series of diagnostic imaging books. This particular title aims to provide an overview and guide to routine mammographic examinations. We aim for this to be an invaluable tool and training aid, a true pocket guide providing essential information for mammographic positioning and technique for mammography practitioners at all levels. It is highly illustrated, with the aim of providing a clear, fast, and reliable source of information promoting patient-centred care.

We hope that this guide will be an essential educational tool for trainees at all levels and for universities delivering mammography education and a convenient clinical guide for practising mammographers, including assistant and associate apprenticeship mammographers.

It has been an absolute pleasure to write this book, not least because of the rewarding experience of sharing knowledge and research from years of experience. It has been a demonstration of the benefits of team working and collaboration of skills and knowledge.

We are most grateful of all to those individuals who have allowed us to share their images; often at an anxious time they gave their generous consent to enable expansion of all our learning. We are very grateful to you all.

"Learning never exhausts the mind"
— Leonardo Da Vinci

Claire Borrelli
Dr Claire Mercer

ACKNOWLEDGEMENTS

We are indebted for the help and advice given by very many colleagues throughout the diagnostic imaging community, with contributions enthusiastically given by sonographers, radiologists, physicists, and lecturers from many health institutions, academic departments, the medical imaging industry, professional bodies, and special interest groups.

Working with Andrea Motta @OmSalvej supported by Studio Salford (https://studio.salford.ac.uk) was an absolute pleasure and truly evidences the benefits of how illustrations can demonstrate practice. We are indebted to you, effortlessly converting our thoughts into these book illustrations; Andrea Motta, thank you so much.

ABBREVIATIONS

2D	Two-dimensional
3D	Three-dimensional
AEC	Automatic exposure control
CB	Core biopsy
CC	Cranio-caudal
CPD	Continuing professional development
CT	Computed tomography
DBT	Digital breast tomosynthesis
FFDM	Full field digital mammography
FNA	Fine needle aspiration
HAI	Healthcare-acquired infection
HCPC	The Health and Care Professions Council
IMF	Infra-mammary fold
MLO	Medio-lateral oblique
MRI	Magnetic resonance imaging
NHSBSP	National Health Service Breast Screening Programme
PPE	Personal protective equipment
RNI	Radionuclide imaging
QA	Quality assurance
QC	Quality control
UK	United Kingdom
WRMSD	Work-related musculo-skeletal disorders

SECTION 1

KEY ASPECTS OF MAMMOGRAPHY PRACTICE

ANATOMY

The breast (mammary gland) is one of the accessory organs of the female reproductive system (**Figure 1.1**). The adult breasts comprise two rounded eminences situated on the anterior and lateral walls of the chest, lying superficially to the pectoral muscles and separated from them by areolar tissue and fascia. They extend from the second to the sixth ribs and from the lateral border of the sternum to the mid-axillary line. The superolateral part is prolonged upwards and laterally towards the axilla to form the axillary tail. The nipple is a conical projection just below the centre of the breast, corresponding approximately to the fourth/fifth intercostal space.[1]

The breast is composed of glandular, fibrous, and fatty tissue. Its size, shape, and consistency vary significantly, depending on the individual's size, shape, and age. Each breast consists of 15–20 lobes, each of which is divided into several lobules. The lobules comprise large numbers of

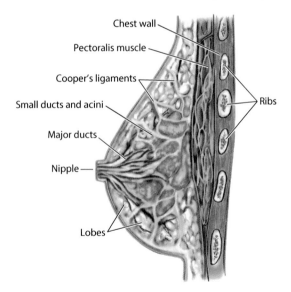

Figure 1.1. Illustration of breast anatomy. (From https://reference.medscape.com/article/1273133-overview. Original source: Wikimedia Commons; Patrick J Lynch. Published under CC BY 2.5 license.)

secretory alveoli, which drain into a single lactiferous duct for each lobe, before converging towards the nipple into the ampullae and opening onto the surface. The blood supply is derived from branches of the axillary, intercostal, and internal mammary arteries. Lymphatic drainage from the breast is primarily via the ipsilateral (same) side.

Axillary lymph nodes (**Figure 1.2**) account for approximately 75% of drainage. The remainder drains via the parasternal and abdominal lymph nodes. It is important to understand lymphatic drainage of the breast as this is the primary route by which breast cancer metastasises (spreads to other parts of the body). Imaging of normal and enlarged lymph nodes is frequently included in the mammographic investigation.[1,2]

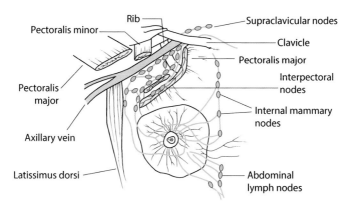

Figure 1.2. Illustration representing lymph drainage. (From https://www.bmj.com/content/309/6963/1222. With permission.)

Breast Tissue Characteristics

With increasing age and especially after the menopause (**Figure 1.3a**), the glandular elements of the breast become less prominent and tend to be replaced by adipose tissue (fat). Fat attenuates the X-ray beam less than glandular breast tissue, as a result the fatty breast is darker. Significant disease (which tends to be dense and produce high attenuation or bright areas on the image) is detected more easily. Younger breast tissue (**Figure 1.3b**) is denser (whiter), and the sensitivity

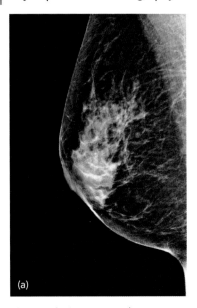
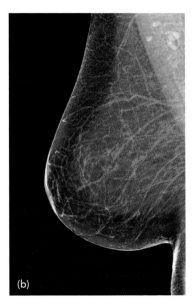

Figure 1.3. Mammography image representing anatomy in (a) younger and (b) older breast tissue. (Reproduced from Whitley et al., 2020.)

(i.e., the ability to detect disease) of mammography in those under 50 years of age is thus reduced. The younger breast is also more sensitive to the adverse effects of ionising radiation. Thus, the reduced sensitivity of mammographic imaging plus the increased radiosensitivity of the breast makes ultrasound the first-line investigation in younger patients, especially less than 35 years of age.[1,2]

Additional Considerations

Mammography is the radiographic examination of the breast tissue (soft tissue radiography). To visualise normal structures and pathology within the breast, it is essential that sharpness, contrast, and resolution are maximised. This optimises, in the image, the relatively small differences in the absorption characteristics of the structures comprising the breast. A low kVp value, typically 28 kVp, is used. Radiation dose must be minimised due to the radiosensitivity of breast tissue.[1–3]

Notes

Mammography is carried out on those who present with a known history or suspected abnormality of the breast, and as a screening procedure in asymptomatic individuals. Consistency of radiographic technique and image quality is essential, particularly in screening mammography, where comparison with previous images is often essential. While other modalities have a role in breast imaging, mammography is undertaken to image the breast most commonly and is hence considered here. Other modalities may be considered for breast imaging – ultrasound, radionuclide imaging (RNI), magnetic resonance imaging (MRI) and computed tomography (CT) – but are not included within this pocketbook for mammography.

POSITIONING TERMINOLOGY

Despite the great individual variation in the external form of the breast, the approximately circular attachment to the chest wall is constant. Vertically, the attachment extends from the second to the sixth rib, and at the level of the fourth costal cartilage it extends transversely from the side of the sternum to the mid-axillary line. A line drawn from the centre of the circle to the nipple can be termed the 'breast axis'. Two planes of importance in radiographic positioning pass through the breast axis. The axial plane divides the breast into inner and outer portions; the transverse plane lies at right angles to the vertical axial plane, intersecting it along the breast axis. The breast is thus divided into quadrants (**Figure 1.4**), termed upper outer, lower outer,

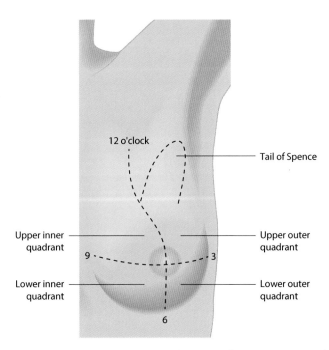

Figure 1.4. Diagram illustrating anatomical aspects of the breast. (Reproduced from Whitley et al., 2020.)

lower inner, and upper inner, respectively. In the normal erect resting position, the axial plane makes an angle of 20–30° with the sagittal plane of the body, and the transverse plane makes an angle of 30–50° with the horizontal.[1]

A prolongation into the axilla of the superolateral portion of the breast along the lower border of pectoralis major is called the axillary tail. The retromammary space lies behind the glandular tissue and should be visible (at least in part) on a correctly positioned mammogram. Microscopically, the breast consists of 15–20 lobes, supported by a stroma of fibrous tissue, which contains a variable quantity of fat. Each lobe has a main duct, opening in the nipple. Deeply, the ducts branch within the breast to drain lobules. Each lobule consists of a cluster of small ductules, into which the glandular epithelium cells pass their secretions. Lobules are demonstrated radiographically as fine, nodular opacities, individually measuring 12 mm in diameter but usually superimposed to give a more or less homogeneous opacity.[1]

With progressive involution (regression of mammary tissue to a non-secreting state), and disappearance of much of the epithelial tissue, the lobules successively shrink and become invisible. Involution commences in the subcutaneous and retromammary regions, then progresses sequentially through the lower inner quadrant, the upper inner and lower outer quadrants, and finally the upper outer quadrant. Involution affects breast density and the ability to handle and position the breast.

Additional Considerations

A young dense breast (i.e., prior to involution) is firmer and less manoeuvrable. Prior to involution in the younger breast, increased density of the tissues can cause further challenges for the practitioner when lifting and positioning the breast tissue away from the chest wall. Compression levels may be compromised, and tolerance of compression could also be affected.

Notes

When considering positioning terminology, the linked nature of the tube and image-recording mechanism make the direction and location of the X-ray beam implicit in the description of the position of the individual and image receptor (**Figure 1.5**).[1]

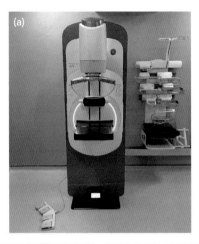

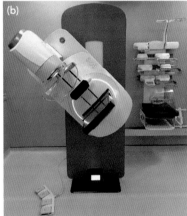
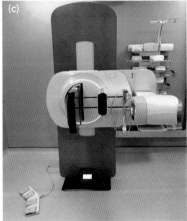

Figure 1.5. Typical mammography equipment with (a) X-ray tube and detector in vertical orientation, (b) X-ray tube and detector in an angled orientation, and (c) X-ray tube and detector in horizontal orientation.

QUALITY CONTROL AND QUALITY ASSURANCE

This is the application of techniques to ensure that a system, or individual, is performing at an optimal level. Quality control (QC) contributes to quality assurance (QA) by ensuring that the equipment, for example the detector, is performing at optimal levels. The performance of the breast imaging service (either breast screening or symptomatic) is dependent on all its integral parts, and no quality assurance initiative should be seen in isolation, even though the performance of each part of the system is measured against a specific stated objective.[1]

It is the responsibility of the employer and the installer of equipment to ensure that quality control tests for the equipment and training for the practitioners undertaking the tests are carried out on all new equipment. The manager, or individual elected responsible by the service, should ensure that the test results are satisfactory and within tolerance levels before the machine is used clinically and that continual testing and audit are undertaken to ensure optimisation of the equipment for service delivery.[2,3]

Responsibilities Within the NHS Breast Screening Programme (NHSBSP)

QA is an intrinsic part of the NHSBSP in maintaining a service which meets national standards and the needs of all individuals invited for screening. There are national guidelines available that provide clear and detailed information on the mammographic aspects (both clinical and technical) of breast screening QA and the QC of radiographic procedures. They:

- provide a framework for auditing, identifying, reporting, and resolving problems;
- drive continuous improvement in quality for all radiographic aspects of breast screening service delivery;
- promote and encourage the development of a learning culture;
- support the promotion of best practice, training, and continuing professional development (CPD).

While QC and QA are mandatory within the NHSBSP, many symptomatic and private sector providers adopt this as best practice to provide a high-quality service.[2]

Responsibilities for QC

All practitioners should ensure that departmental protocols for routine QC are developed and followed. Written operational procedures for the routine monitoring, testing, and servicing of equipment must be approved by the local QA medical physicist. Practitioners should be involved in equipment specification and selection, acceptance, and commissioning testing, and in service testing.

The quality of mammography depends on the expertise of practitioners as well as on the performance of equipment. Each department must have a method of recording test results to ensure that the information is evaluated and monitored, and that corrective action is taken and recorded. A document control system must be used for all written procedures and forms.

The QC system and the results produced should be regularly reviewed and modified as necessary considering changing knowledge and experience.

The objectives are to achieve optimum image quality with as low a radiation dose as practicable. The achievement of these objectives requires mammographers, medical physics services, and service personnel to work closely together.[3]

Additional Considerations

Practitioners have a responsibility for regular audit of their clinical practice to maintain high-quality breast imaging and clinical competence. Limiting repeat examinations, they should review their own performance against personal, department/unit, regional, and national standards, as appropriate by the employer. This may identify equipment problems or indicate a training need.

Notes

Mammographic QC in a department is the responsibility of all mammographers and is monitored by the superintendent/manager (or the named QC mammographer). The role of a QC mammographer is to:[1,2]

- oversee the monitoring of mammographic image quality in the department; this should be both educational and developmental;
- monitor technical repeat examinations, audit the findings, and take appropriate action where necessary;
- ensure compliance with radiographic QC guidelines;
- liaise with medical physics and discuss outcomes of equipment testing;
- know who is responsible for authorisation of suspension from use of equipment when tolerances are exceeded and understand the procedure for taking action;
- maintain strong links with the local and regional QA network;
- identify their own educational and development needs through appraisal and a development review process and seek to address those needs;
- work in conjunction with the health and safety representative, to assist mammography practitioners to work in an environment conducive to their health and welfare;
- understand the process for highlighting and resolving system failures.

COMMUNICATION AND CONSENT

Prior to any mammographic examination, informed choice and informed consent must be obtained from the individual.[1,4]

Informed Consent to Mammography

An explanation of the mammographic procedure before it is performed must include the use and implications of radiation and compression. For consent to be valid, it must be given voluntarily (without pressure from others), as part of an informed choice, and the individual must have the capacity to consent. Capacity means the individual can understand and use information about the procedure, including benefits and risks. It is the practitioner's professional judgement to decide whether consent has been given prior to, and maintained throughout, the examination.[2,4]

The legal and professional frameworks in informed choice and consent are subject to change; practitioners have a professional responsibility to keep their knowledge up to date in all areas of their practice (HCPC standards). If consent is not given freely and is not in place, the examination must not be undertaken.[1]

Additional Considerations

- If the individual expresses any apprehension or uncertainties about having breast imaging performed, the practitioner should do everything possible to sensitively address those concerns at the time.
- If consent is withdrawn at any stage, the examination must be stopped, and cessation of the examination documented.
- Postponement of an appointment to allow the individual time to consider whether to attend may be appropriate.
- The limitations of mammography in the presence of breast implants or medical implanted devices must be explained fully prior to undertaking any imaging. This may impact on the individual's decision to give consent.

Notes

Associate/Assistant practitioners who are trained via an accredited or approved academic programme and are competency-assessed may take consent to mammography as one of the responsibilities delegated to them by registered radiographers. However, this is limited to those who are cooperative and able to communicate their consent. If consent is in doubt, the supervising registered radiographer must be consulted.[2,4]

Note should also be given to the role that privacy and confidentiality may play in achieving consent from the individual prior to the examination. Practitioners must ensure that they undertake information governance training and act in accordance with the local employer protocols.

WORK-RELATED MUSCULO-SKELETAL DISORDERS (WRMSD)

Due to the repetitive nature of breast imaging and the fact that undertaking a mammogram is a notably physical activity, great care should be taken to support the well-being of mammography staff. Common areas of the body to be affected by musculo-skeletal pain for practitioners include the hands, wrists, elbows, shoulders, neck, and lower back, although this list is not exclusive[1] (**Figure 1.6**).

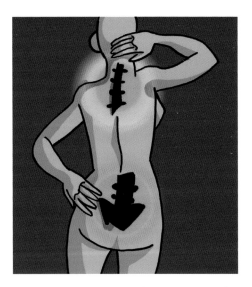

Figure 1.6. Diagrammatic representation of common areas of the body to be affected by musculo-skeletal pain.

Responsibility

It is the responsibility of individuals to adopt best practice for their own health and safety and that of work colleagues to ensure that safe practices are used when performing mammography and undertaking other imaging-related duties. The health and safety of all practitioners performing mammograms are critically important, and the Employers' Liability Act makes it the employer's responsibility to care for the health and safety of their employees while at work.[5] From an occupational health perspective, prevention is more effective than treatment for WRMSD.

With the increasing workload in breast imaging and the requirement to maintain constantly high-quality imaging to aid cancer detection, practitioners are likely to adopt unusual postures when pressed for time, although positioning should ideally be efficient and timely to reduce the risk of injury.[5]

Ergonomic recommendations for the management team to consider limiting the effects of WRMSD should include consideration of the following:

- room size and design, equipment;
- schedule of appointments;
- staff rotation and working patterns.

A risk assessment should be undertaken to identify sensible measures to control risk in the workplace. Ergonomic recommendations for the individual will include awareness of areas prone to work-related injury, and awareness of research and guidance documents to promote good ergonomic practice.[5,6]

Best Practice

It is important to identify alternative postures for practitioners while performing mammography, which can help to reduce the risk of WRMSD. Good communication with the individual will enable them to move independently rather than be moved by the practitioner and reduce the potential for discomfort or potential injury.

Practitioners should make sure they are familiar with the location of X-ray unit controls, so they do not overstretch unnecessarily. They should try not to use the same fingers to press the exposure button. Different exposure control designs exist, involving different types of movement. Selecting an appropriate means of control can avoid injury.[1]

Before positioning an individual, it should be ensured that the foot pedals are placed correctly so there is no need to stretch extremities. A seated position for the examination could be considered, both for the individual and the practitioner. This will require suitable aids and flooring. Each practitioner must adjust their seat height and proximity to suit each individual, and each should avoid overextension of their elbows and shoulders. The wheels on the stool must be selected to give the right level of grip for the type of floor (**Figure 1.7a,b**). Between

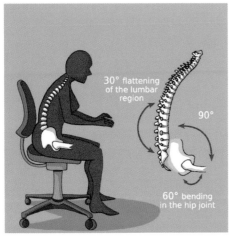

30° flattening of the lumbar region

90°

60° bending in the hip joint

Conventional sitting in a 90/90 degree angle can cause many chronic health problems.

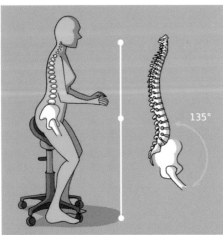

135°

On a divided saddle chair, a good and healthy posture can be maintained automatically, if the chair is used correctly.

Figure 1.7. Diagrammatic representation of (a) conventional and (b) suggested seating in a saddle chair to support healthy posture.

16

individuals, the practitioner could alternate starting position from seated to standing to reduce repetition where possible.[1]

When positioning an individual, the whole hand, or as much of the hand as possible, should be used to position the breast, rather than relying on the thumb and forefinger. Unnecessary use of manual hand compression controls should be avoided to prevent wrist strain (**Figure 1.8**).

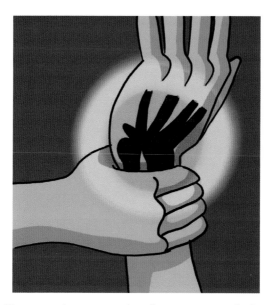

Figure 1.8. Diagrammatic representation of common areas of wrist strain.

Additional Considerations

Where possible, the height of the modality acquisition workstation should be set. Some manufacturers have introduced touchscreen technology to reduce the use of keyboards.

Two practitioners should be available when individuals with additional needs (e.g., an individual in a wheelchair) are attending for mammography.

Observation of colleagues and offering feedback to correct poor technique and poor adoption of posture is valuable and should be seen as good practice.

Additional equipment should be stored at waist height to reduce bending and stretching.

Notes

To reduce WRMSD, the Health and Safety Executive recommends that employees complete exercises before the start of the working day and during their micro-breaks between examinations. Employees may want to seek guidance from occupational health colleagues.

WORKING PRACTICES

Infection prevention and control is the use of safe practices and ways of working that help to prevent or reduce infections within healthcare settings. Good standards of infection prevention and control are essential to safeguard the health and safety of all individuals, members of the public, and staff, and are a legal duty of hospitals. All staff hold a responsibility to have a working knowledge and demonstrate compliance with employer and government guidelines for infection prevention and control.[7,8] The hospital may be served an improvement service notice for breaches in standards.[9] Mammography departments could consider the development of a link practitioner role to the infection control team to support the provision of current advice and guidance regarding infection control.[10]

Standard Precautions

Standard precautions consist of the following:[1,11]

- correct hand hygiene;
- safe use of personal protective equipment (PPE), which may include gloves, impermeable gowns, plastic aprons, masks, face shields, and eye protection;
- safe handling of blood and body fluids;
- sharps safety;
- safe cleaning and decontamination;
- environmental cleanliness;
- safe handling and disposal of waste and linen;
- respiratory hygiene.

To Reduce Preventable Infections

Healthcare-acquired infections (HAIs) are infections that are contracted as a direct result of treatment or contact in a healthcare setting,[11] but many are preventable. Staying well informed regarding the latest guidance on the spread of infections and strategies for prevention is essential for a successful infection prevention programme. Key work instructions/protocols to read and demonstrate compliance if working in the healthcare setting include:

- Hand Hygiene Protocol;
- Personal Protective Equipment (PPE) Policy;[7]
- Glove Policy;
- Safe Use and Disposal of Sharps;
- Sharps Injury and Splash;
- Decontamination Policy;
- Dress Code Policy.

Under Breast Soreness – Intertrigo

Some individuals will have a rash under their breasts or between some of the folds in their skin. This is often caused by a common skin condition called intertrigo, the main causes of which are moisture, heat, and friction between skin folds. The practitioner can often find the individual's skin raw, cracked, and weeping. As a practitioner great care must be taken when positioning for a mammogram to avoid tearing this fragile skin.[11]

Additional Considerations

The identified SARS-CoV-2 virus with the associated disease COVID-19 began a pandemic in 2019. This brought additional considerations and guidance for staff working in healthcare settings, which saw considerable changes to what is now standard practice. All healthcare employers have a responsibility to comply with the most up-to-date government guidelines and ensure that all staff have access to and abide by the guidelines to reduce the spread of infections within the workplace.[10,11]

Consideration should also be given to the importance of care and cleaning of equipment and the environment in which it is sited. Local protocols should be adhered to, to ensure and promote safe practice. Where mobile units may be used for remote service delivery, consideration of mobile design and resuming service provision after a prolonged pause, may also be helpful.[12]

Notes

All healthcare regulators have a responsibility to monitor, inspect, and regulate services to ensure they meet the fundamental standards of quality and safety, and to publish what they find, including performance ratings, to help people choose care. Regulators are required to set out what good and outstanding care looks like and to ensure services meet fundamental standards below which care must never fall.

BREAST COMPRESSION

Essential Considerations

The breast is compressed to a level that can be tolerated by the individual within the required standards: between 9 and 13 daN,[13] and remaining under the maximum level of 20 daN.[11,13–15] It is important to ensure standardisation of breast thickness/compression level for an individual at each attendance. This is to enable a consistent experience and to produce mammography images that can be compared at each attendance.[16]

For compression application the practitioner can operate the remote-controlled foot compression device, or the individual can control the hand-held compression device (under the supervision of the practitioner) if available on the equipment. Extreme care must be taken when the compression is applied to ensure that exposure is imminent, ensuring the individual remains under compression for the minimal time. Compression must be released as soon as the exposure ends. It is important that the breast is positioned optimally, or compression will be unnecessarily painful and may cause a reduction in repeat participation of breast cancer screening.[17–20]

Additional Considerations

The amount of pressure exerted on the individual's breast is the amount of force applied to the breast tissue divided by the area of the breast tissue being compressed. So, a smaller-breasted individual would receive a higher pressure than a larger-breasted individual for the same amount of force applied – this could cause an unnecessary amount of discomfort with no additional benefit to quality.[11,19,20]

Notes

It is important that the breast is positioned optimally, or compression will be unnecessarily uncomfortable.

Standardise compression (10 kPa with a range of 7–15 kPa) for an individual to enable a consistent experience and to produce mammography images that are comparable between screening attendances.

REFERENCES

1. Whitley, S.A., Dodgeon, J., Meadows, A., Cullingworth, J., Holmes, K., Jackson, M., Hoadley, G., and Kulshrestha, R. *Clark's Procedures in Diagnostic Imaging: A System-Based Approach*. CRC Press, 2020.
2. Public Health England. Breast screening: guidance for breast screening mammographers. 2020. Available at: https://www.gov.uk/government/publications/breast-screening-quality-assurance-for-mammography-and-radiography.
3. The Royal College of Radiologists. IR(ME)R: Implications for clinical practice in diagnostic imaging, interventional radiology and diagnostic nuclear medicine. BFCR(20)3. 2020. Available at: https://www.rcr.ac.uk/publication/irmer-implications-diagnostic-imaging-interventional-radiology-diagnostic-nuclear-medicine.
4. The Society of Radiographers. Obtaining consent: a clinical guideline for the diagnostic imaging and radiotherapy workforce. 2020. Available at: https://www.sor.org/learning-advice/professional-body-guidance-and-publications/documents-and-publications/policy-guidance-document-library/obtaining-consent-a-clinical-guideline-for-the-dia.
5. HM Government. The Employers Liability Act. 1969. Available at: https://www.legislation.gov.uk/ukpga/1969/57/contents.
6. Public Health England. Breast screening mammography: ergonomics good practice. 2018. Available at: https://www.gov.uk/government/publications/breast-screening-ergonomics-in-screening-mammography/breast-screening-mammography-ergonomics-good-practice.
7. Health and Safety Executive. Personal protective equipment (PPE) at work regulations from 6 April 2022. Available at: https://www.hse.gov.uk/ppe/ppe-regulations-2022.htm.
8. NHS England. National infection prevention and control. 2022. Available at: https://www.england.nhs.uk/publication/national-infection-prevention-and-control.
9. Health and Social Care Act 2012. Available at: https://www.legislation.gov.uk/ukpga/2012/7/contents/enacted.
10. National Institute for Health and Care Excellence (NICE). Healthcare-associated infections: prevention and control [PH36]. 2011. Available at: https://www.nice.org.uk/guidance/ph36.
11. Mercer, C., Hogg, P., and Kelly, J. *Digital Mammography: A Holistic Approach*. 2nd edition. UK: Springer, 2022.

12. National Co-ordinating Centre for the Physics of Mammography (NCCPM). Advice on care and maintenance of NHS Breast Screening Programme mammography equipment and trailers when not in use over a prolonged period. 2020. Available at: https://medphys. royalsurrey.nhs.uk/nccpm/files/other/Advice-X-ray-equipment-V11b.pdf.

13. Hogg, P., Taylor, M., Szczepura, K., Mercer, C., and Denton, E. Pressure and breast thickness in mammography—an exploratory calibration study. *The British Journal of Radiology* 2013;**86**(1021):20120222. https://doi.org/10.1259/bjr.20120222.

14. Smith, H., Szczepura, K., Mercer, C., Maxwell, A., and Hogg, P. Does elevating image receptor increase breast receptor footprint and improve pressure balance? *Radiography* 2015;**21**(4):359–363. https:// doi.org/10.1016/j.radi.2015.02.001.

15. European Commission Initiative on Breast Cancer. European guidelines on breast cancer screening and diagnosis. 2021. Available at: https://healthcare-quality.jrc.ec.europa.eu/ecibc/ european-breast-cancer-guidelines.

16. Whelehan, P., Evans, A., Wells, M., and Macgillivray, S. The effect of mammography pain on repeat participation in breast cancer screening: a systematic review. *Breast* 2013;**22**(4):389–394.

17. Agius, E.C., and Naylor, S. Breast compression techniques in screening mammography – a Maltese evaluation project. *Radiography* 2018;**24**(4):309–314.

18. Moshina, N., Bjørnson, E.W., Holen, Å.S., Larsen, M., Hansestad, B., Tøsdal, L., and Hofvind, S. Standardised or individualised X-ray tube angle for mediolateral oblique projection in digital mammography? *Radiography* 2022;**28**(3):772–778.

19. De Groot, J.E., Broeders, M.J.M., Branderhorst, W., den Heeten, G.J., and Grimbergen, C.A. A novel approach to mammographic breast compression: improved standardization and reduced discomfort by controlling pressure instead of force. *Medical Physics* 2013;**40**(8):081901.

20. Branderhorst, W., de Groot, J.E., Neeter, L.M., van Lier, M.G., Neeleman, C., den Heeten, G.J., et al. Force balancing in mammographic compression. *Medical Physics* 2016;**43**(1):518.

SECTION 2

ROUTINE MAMMOGRAPHIC PROJECTIONS

ROUTINE PROJECTIONS: CRANIO-CAUDAL (CC)

This projection demonstrates the majority of the breast, excluding the superior posterior portion, the axillary tail, and the extreme medial portion, which contains less glandular tissue than the lateral portion.[1] The projection is described with the individual standing but can be achieved with the individual seated or in a wheelchair.

Position of the Individual and Image Receptor

The individual faces the mammography equipment, which is pointing vertically downwards, with arms by their sides and feet facing forwards, stood slightly back from the image receptor (**Figure 2.1**).

Their head is turned away from the side under examination, and the shoulder on the side under examination is dropped to promote coverage of the lateral posterior portion of the breast. This will bring the outer quadrant of their breast in contact with the image receptor and relax the pectoral muscle.[1] The image receptor is positioned at the level of their infra-mammary fold (IMF).

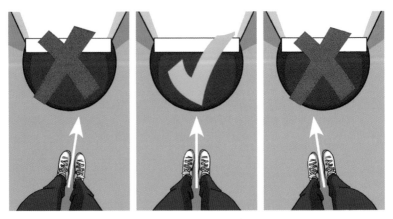

Figure 2.1 Position of the individual's feet in relation to the image receptor. (Modified from Mercer et al., 2022. With permission.)

The practitioner stands on the side that is not being examined and lifts the individual's breast up in the palm of their hand. The image receptor will then need to be raised slightly to lift the breast above the level of the IMF by around 1–2 cm to ensure even distribution of pressure across the breast tissue.[2] Care must be taken to ensure the height of the image receptor optimises the maximum amount of breast tissue on the image receptor, while ensuring the nipple remains in the midline of the detector and in profile[2,3] (**Figure 2.2**).

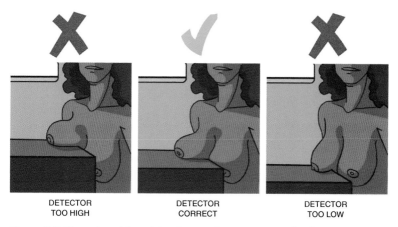

| DETECTOR TOO HIGH | DETECTOR CORRECT | DETECTOR TOO LOW |

Figure 2.2 Correct position of the detector/image receptor for the cranio-caudal position. The left diagram demonstrates the position being too high, while the right diagram demonstrates the position being too low. (Modified from Mercer et al., 2022. With permission.)

The position of the breast should then be checked to ensure that the nipple remains in profile (**Figure 2.3**).

The breast is compressed to a level that can be tolerated within the required standards: between 9 and 13 daN,[3] and remaining under the maximum level of 20 daN.[4–6] It is important to ensure standardisation of breast thickness/compression level for each individual at each attendance. This is to enable a consistent experience and to produce mammography images that can be compared at each attendance.[6]

Compression must be released as soon as the exposure ends. It is important that the breast must be positioned optimally, or compression

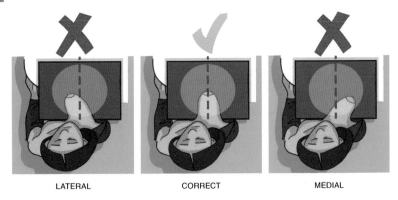

| LATERAL | CORRECT | MEDIAL |

Figure 2.3 Correct position of the nipple in the cranio-caudal position. The left diagram illustrates that the breast needs to be laterally rotated, while the right diagram illustrates that the breast needs to be medially rotated. (Modified from Mercer et al., 2022. With permission.)

will be unnecessarily painful and may cause a reduction in repeat participation of breast cancer screening.[7,8]

Essential Image Characteristics

The images should be symmetrical with adequate compression (**Figure 2.4**) to hold the breast in position with no movement, demonstrating the:

- medial and lateral borders;
- posterior aspect of the breast;
- some of the axillary tail;
- pectoral muscle shadow;
- nipple in profile and shown to the midline of the image;
- no skin folds in the breast tissue or artefacts obscuring the image.

Additional Considerations

The nipple should be demonstrated in at least one view (CC and/or MLO). It may not be in profile due to incorrect image receptor height:[1]

- if too low, the nipple will be tilted below the breast tissue;
- if too high, the nipple will lie above the breast tissue.

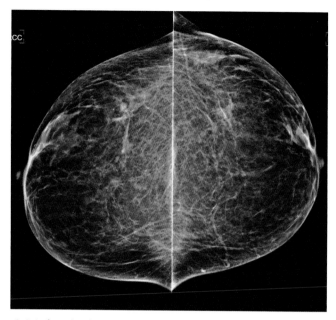

Figure 2.4 Left and right cranio-caudal mammography images. (Reproduced from Whitley et al., 2020.)

Occasionally the skin on the underside of the breast can be caught in the IMF.

A supplementary projection of this area is essential if the nipple is not in profile, if no improvement can be made without the loss of visualisation of breast tissue and there is not a clear representation on the MLO projection.[1,5] This may be due to factors outside of the individual and the practitioners' control, for example, previous surgery.

Notes

- Automatic exposure controls are used for standard/routine mammography.
- If imaging implants or medical devices, settings will have to be adjusted.

ROUTINE PROJECTIONS: MEDIO-LATERAL OBLIQUE (MLO)

This projection demonstrates the greatest amount of breast tissue of any single projection. In a complete breast examination, there must be visually sharp reproduction of the whole glandular breast, visually sharp reproduction of the cutaneous and subcutaneous tissue, and the nipple should be parallel to the image receptor.[4,5] The projection is described with the individual standing but can be achieved with the individual seated or in a wheelchair.

Position of the Individual and Image Receptor

It is important to recognise that every individual is different, starting with the angle of the mammography system around 45° or 50°, the

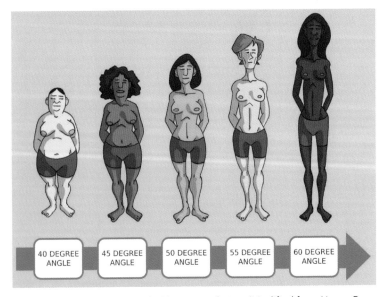

Figure 2.5 Initial medio-lateral oblique angulation. (Modified from Hogg, P., Kelly, J., and Mercer, C. *Digital Mammography: A Holistic Approach*. 2015. London: Springer. With permission.)

practitioner will then adapt to the angle of the individual's body habitus and height[3,7,9–12] (**Figure 2.5**). This is important to ensure high-quality images are achieved with minimal radiation dose and minimal discomfort to the individual.

The individual faces the equipment, with their feet apart for stability and the lateral edge of their rib cage in line with the image receptor. It is at this point that the image receptor angle can be adjusted to align with the individual[1,6] (**Figure 2.6**).

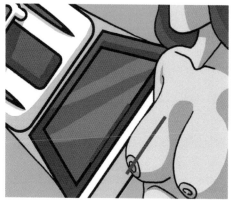

Figure 2.6 Medio-lateral oblique angulation adjustment. (Modified from Mercer et al., 2022. With permission.)

With the individual's arm placed on the top of the image receptor platform, their elbow flexed and relaxed behind it (**Figure 2.7a and b**), the image receptor height is adjusted so that the lower border of the breast is around 2–3 cm above the edge of the image receptor.[1] The individual's breast is bought forwards and gently extended upwards and outwards to ensure it contacts the image receptor. By leaning the individual forwards, the shoulder on the side of examination is then lifted and extended to ensure inclusion of the axilla, the axillary tail, and as much as possible of the breast tissue.[1]

The practitioner maintains an upward and outward lift on the breast under examination, while the other hand gently removes any skin folds, especially between the lateral aspect of the breast and the image

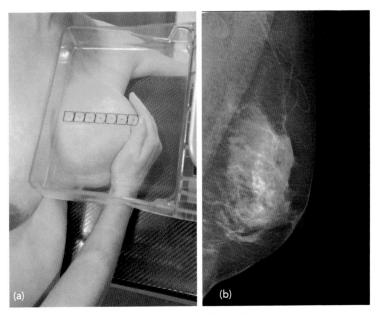

Figure 2.7 (a) Positioning for medio-lateral oblique. (b) Image of medio-lateral oblique projection. (Reproduced from Whitley et al., 2020.)

receptor behind it. Compression is applied, ensuring this fits the angle of the humeral head and the chest wall. Great care must be taken not to cause pain to the individual, commonly around the ribs or sternum. During the initial application of compression, a slight movement away of the opposite side of the individual's body is required until the compression paddle touches the breast under examination, then the individual can be rotated back inwards. When the compression is almost complete, the practitioner removes their hand and undertakes a final check for skin folds; premature removal will cause the breast to droop.[1]

The breast is compressed to a level that can be tolerated within the required standards, between 9 and 13 daN,[3] and remaining under the maximum level of 20 daN.[4–6] It is important to ensure standardisation of breast thickness/compression level for each individual at each attendance to enable a consistent experience and to produce mammography images that can be compared on each attendance.[5]

Compression must be released as soon as the exposure ends. It is important to note that the breast must be positioned optimally, or compression will be unnecessarily painful and may influence repeat participation in breast cancer screening.[7,8]

Essential Image Characteristics

The images should be symmetrical (**Figure 2.8**) with adequate compression to hold the breast firmly in position with no movement and demonstrate:

- axilla, axillary tail, glandular tissue, pectoral muscle, and IMF;
- pectoral muscle at an appropriate angle across the image between 20° and 35°;
- nipple in profile and shown to the midline of the image; normally will be demonstrated in at least one view (CC and/or MLO);
- no skin folds in the breast tissue or overlying structures/artefacts obscuring the image.

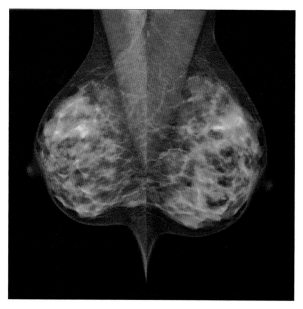

Figure 2.8 Left and right medio-lateral oblique mammography images. (Reproduced from Whitley et al., 2020.)

Additional Considerations

If the axillary area is not clearly demonstrated, the image receptor was too low – ensure that the nipple is one-third of the way up the image receptor.

If the pectoral muscle is not clearly demonstrated, this is due to the individual not leaning in towards the image receptor and not extending the arm and shoulder up and over the image receptor adequately.

Not all the breast tissue may be demonstrated due to incorrect positioning; this can be rectified in the following situations:

- Lack of IMF: stand the individual further forwards from the image receptor.
- Missing inferior aspect of the breast: align the individual's feet and hips with the rest of their body.
- Missing lower border of the breast on the image: lower the image receptor height or ensure not to release the breast prior to adequate compression application.
- Nipple not in profile: ensure the individual's body is parallel with the image receptor. If too far forward, the nipple will rotate under the breast tissue; too far back and the nipple will lie above the midline and not all the breast tissue will be demonstrated.

Notes

- Usually, automatic exposure controls are used for standard/routine mammography.
- If imaging implants or medical devices, settings will have to be adjusted.
- The decision of whether or not to perform repeat imaging should be taken according to specific department protocols and ionising radiation regulations.

TOMOSYNTHESIS

Digital breast tomosynthesis or DBT is a technique of 3D breast imaging. Many images are acquired of a compressed breast, at multiple angles (**Figure 2.9**), and then reconstructed for viewing. Conventional mammography is a 2D imaging modality, thus, on occasion, pathologies can be masked or misinterpreted due to overlying structures. DBT aims to overcome or reduce this overlap effect by acquiring images at numerous different angles. The data can then be reconstructed to display individual slices or as a moving cine image.

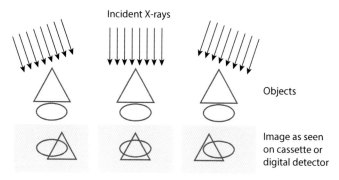

Figure 2.9 Diagrammatic representation of tomosynthesis image. (Reproduced from Whitley et al., 2020.)

Positioning of the Individual and Image Receptor

Careful explanations are required to ensure compliance, as the exposure time, and therefore compression, is slightly longer than for conventional mammography. The individual will be positioned as for one or both routine mammography projections – MLO and CC. Image acquisition will follow a standard protocol determined by the equipment manufacturer. This may include:

- Select appropriate individual demographics from the worklist or manual data entry.

- Select appropriate protocol from the database.
- Position the individual, mammography tube, and image receptor (**Figure 2.10a**).
- Take a scout acquisition to confirm positioning, collimation, and technique; multiple scouts may be taken for better positioning or improved technical parameters.
- Auto-position the mammography tube to the start position.
- Press and hold the exposure button until the sweep has finished and acquisitions are complete (**Figure 2.10b**).

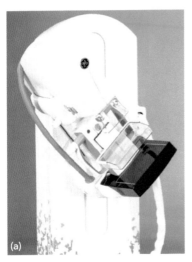

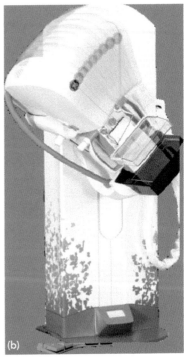

Figure 2.10 Diagrammatic representation of equipment stationary (a) and moving (b). (Reproduced from Whitley et al., 2020.)

Essential Image Characteristics

This will be as described for the routine projections for the CC and MLO.

Additional Considerations

As having DBT takes a little longer than a standard mammogram, with both CC and MLO images taken, the breast will be compressed for a longer timeframe but slightly less compression is required.

The use of 2D full field digital mammography (FFDM) images plus 3D DBT images in both projections is controversial and not currently acceptable in routine breast screening. This may be overcome by reconstructing the 2D image from the 3D dataset, producing a synthetic 2D image.

DBT may be used within the symptomatic services and private provider services.

Notes

A trial in the UK NHS Breast Screening Programme compared DBT with digital mammography.[13] The trial concluded that while specificity improved with DBT and 2D, over 2D alone, sensitivity improved only marginally. Further, it was stated that synthetic 2D appeared to be comparable with standard 2D, and the authors recommended further study to compare 2D and synthetic 2D for different lesion types.

DBT may well replace conventional 2D FFDM in the future, specifically in personalised screening for those at high risk, including those with dense breast parenchyma.

THE AUGMENTED BREAST

As breast implants are radio-opaque, visualisation of breast tissue is often not possible and this presents an important imaging challenge for the practitioner. Those with breast implants who attend for mammography need to be made aware of the limited nature of the mammographic examination performed on them and a policy should be followed by the imaging department.[14] Breast awareness is vital for those with breast implants.

The anatomical placement of the breast implant is typically subglandular or submuscular (**Figure 2.11**). Implants that are placed below the pectoral muscle may be less likely to interfere with mammography imaging.[15]

HOW BREAST IMPLANTS WORK
SUBGLANDULAR IMPLANT

HOW BREAST IMPLANTS WORK
SUBMUSCULAR IMPLANT

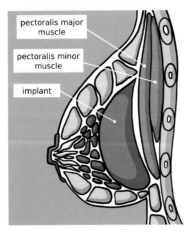

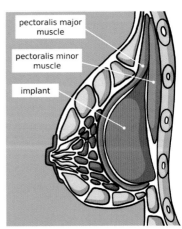

The implant is inserted over both the pectoralis minor and the pectoralis major muscles in the chest.

The implant is fully inserted under the pectoralis major muscle and above the pectoralis minor muscle.

Figure 2.11 Illustration of positioning of breast implants.

Positioning of the Individual and Image Receptor

Using the standard technique, the MLO projection is undertaken first to identify the position of the implant; this may help with decisions about imaging of that individual. The breast is positioned routinely; however, only minimal compression is applied, to a point at which the breast will be held in position (around 4–5 daN).

A manual exposure must be set, as the automatic exposure control (AEC) device would not terminate the exposure due to the radio-opacity of the breast. Guidance is provided by each manufacturer. The resultant mammogram is evaluated particularly with respect to exposure factors and repeated if necessary.

The CC projection is then taken to get as far back onto the chest wall as possible and demonstrate both medial and lateral borders. An additional CC view is then undertaken employing the Eklund or displacement technique to demonstrate the anterior breast tissue with the implant displaced posteriorly.[16]

These views are achieved by pulling breast tissue forward, away from the implant. At the same time, the implant is displaced posteriorly against the chest wall so that it is out of the field of view. The practitioner then applies compression force to the tissue in front of the implant (**Figure 2.12**).

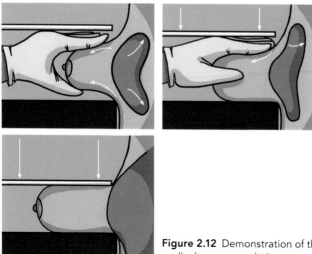

Figure 2.12 Demonstration of the Eklund or displacement technique.

Essential Image Characteristics

Standard CC and MLO views are typically taken first. The implant displacement view, which may also be recognised as the 'push-back technique' (Eklund), provides improved imaging of the tissue at the front of the implant, while the standard views provide images of the tissue behind and underneath the implant, as well as the lower axillary area.[15]

Additional Considerations

It is important to explain clearly to individuals the need for additional images to be able to visualise as much breast tissue as possible to increase sensitivity. Understanding the need for additional imaging will promote informed consent.

In addition, the importance of appropriate communication should be considered. For example, saying "I will ease the breast tissue forward and away from the implant" rather than "I will push the implant back against your chest wall". The choice of terminology may have an impact on the individual.

Injectable fillers may be used for volume restoration and body contouring as an alternative to breast augmentation with implants. Prior to breast imaging, it is useful for the practitioner to know whether breast fillers or fat transfer have been used, as some products may compromise the visualisation of breast tissue and reduce the diagnostic quality of the resultant images.[16,17]

Notes

Tangential projections should be undertaken in those with breast implants and those undergoing mammography due to a localised breast lump.

The Eklund technique[16] is suitable for those in whom there is a large volume of breast tissue relative to the prosthesis, or for those who have had their prosthesis positioned within the glandular tissue and in front of the pectoral muscle (subglandular implant). The implant is displaced (pushed back) to the back of the breast while the natural breast tissue is stretched forward onto the image receptor plate so that only the breast tissue is compressed and imaged (**Figure 2.13**).[1]

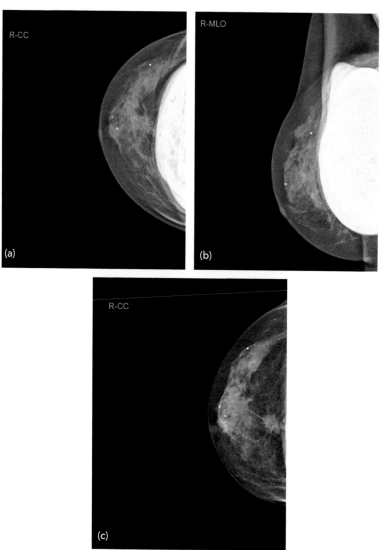

Figure 2.13 (a) Routine cranio-caudal image showing appearance of a breast implant. (b) Routine medio-lateral oblique image showing an augmented breast showing 'push-back' technique. (c) Cranio-caudal image demonstrating a cancer previously obscured by an implant. (Reproduced from Whitley et al., 2020.)

REFERENCES

1. Whitley, S.A., Dodgeon, J., Meadows, A., Cullingworth, J., Holmes, K., Jackson, M., Hoadley, G., and Kulshrestha, R. *Clark's Procedures in Diagnostic Imaging: A System-Based Approach*. CRC Press, 2020.

2. Smith, H., Szczepura, K., Mercer, C., Maxwell, A., and Hogg, P. Does elevating image receptor increase breast receptor footprint and improve pressure balance? *Radiography* 2015;21(4):359–363. https://doi.org/10.1016/j.radi.2015.02.001

3. Hogg, P., Taylor, M., Szczepura, K., Mercer, C., and Denton, E. Pressure and breast thickness in mammography—an exploratory calibration study. *The British Journal of Radiology* 2013;86(1021):20120222. https://www.birpublications.org/doi/10.1259/bjr.20120222

4. European Commission Initiative on Breast Cancer. European guidelines on breast cancer screening and diagnosis. 2021. Available at: https://healthcare-quality.jrc.ec.europa.eu/ecibc/european-breast-cancer-guidelines.

5. Public Health England. Breast screening: guidance for breast screening mammographers. 2020. Available at: https://www.gov.uk/government/publications/breast-screening-quality-assurance-for-mammography-and-radiography.

6. Mercer, C., Szczepura, K., Hill, C.A., Kinnear, L.A., Kelly, A., and Smith, H.L. Practical Mammography. In: Mercer, C., Hogg, P. and Kelly, J. (eds) *Digital Mammography*. Springer, Cham. 2022. https://doi.org/10.1007/978-3-031-10898-3_27.

7. Whelehan, P., Evans, A., Wells, M., and Macgillivray, S. The effect of mammography pain on repeat participation in breast cancer screening: a systematic review. *Breast* 2013;22(4):389–394.

8. Agius, E.C., and Naylor, S. Breast compression techniques in screening mammography – a Maltese evaluation project. *Radiography* 2018;24(4):309–314.

9. Bedene, A., Alukié, E., Žibert, J., and Mekiš, N. Mediolateral oblique projection in mammography: use of different angulation for patients with different thorax anatomies. *Journal of Health Sciences* 2019;9(1):40–45.

10. Moshina, N., Bjørnson, E.W., Holen, Å.S., Larsen, M., Hansestad, B., Tøsdal, L., and Hofvind, S., 2022. Standardised or individualised X-ray tube angle for mediolateral oblique projection in digital mammography? *Radiography* 2022;28(3):772–778.

11. De Groot, J.E., Broeders, M.J.M., Branderhorst, W., den Heeten, G.J., and Grimbergen, C.A. A novel approach to mammographic breast compression: improved standardization and reduced discomfort by controlling pressure instead of force. *Medical Physics* 2013;**40**(8):081901.

12. Branderhorst, W., de Groot, J.E., Neeter, L.M., van Lier, M.G., Neeleman, C., den Heeten, G.J., et al. Force balancing in mammographic compression. *Medical Physics* 2016;**43**(1):518.

13. Gilbert, F., Tucker, L., Gillan, M., et al. The TOMMY trial: A comparison of TOMosynthesis with digital MammographY in the UK NHS Breast Screening Programme. Health Technology Assessment 2015;**19**(4):i–xxv, 1–136.

14. Public Health England. NHS Breast Screening Programme: Screening women with breast implants. Available at: https://assets.publishing. service.gov.uk/government/uploads/system/upload/attachment_ data/file/624796/Screening_women_with_breast_implants_guidance.pdf.

15. Handel, N., Silverstein, M.J., Gamagami, P., Jensen, J.A., and Collins, A. Factors affecting mammographic visualization of the breast after augmentation mammaplasty. *JAMA* 1992;**268**:1913–1917.

16. Eklund, G.W., Busby, R.C., Miller, S.H., and Job, J.S. Improved imaging of the augmented breast. *AJR American Journal of Roentgenology* 1988;**151**:469–473.

17. Ishii, H., and Sakata, K. Complications and management of breast enhancement using hyaluronic acid. *Plastic Surgery* 2014;**22**(3):171–174.

SECTION 3
ADDITIONAL/MODIFIED MAMMOGRAPHIC PROJECTIONS

ADDITIONAL/MODIFIED PROJECTION: CRANIO-CAUDAL – LATERALLY ROTATED

This extended cranio-caudal (CC) projection is useful for demonstrating the outer quadrant, axillary tail, and axilla.[1]

Position of the Individual and Image Receptor

The individual faces the equipment and the side under examination is rotated towards the mammography equipment, their breast is elevated to form a right angle with the body with the nipple in profile. The image receptor is raised to contact the inferior part of the breast closest to the chest wall.[1]

The practitioner places the individual's breast with the nipple area on the extreme medial edge of the image receptor; the individual's arm resting on the side of the equipment. Standing behind the individual, their breast is lifted and extended as far as possible. The individual will lean around 45° back, depressing their shoulder to enable the outer quadrant and axilla to contact the image receptor. With their arm extended, they hold the equipment for stability and to maintain their position.[1]

While the breast is held in position, the individual is asked to lean towards the equipment; it is important to ensure that the nipple is kept in profile. The breast is supported manually while the compression is initiated. The compression paddle will fit into the angle between the humeral head and the rib cage (**Figure 3.1a**).[1]

Great care must be taken not to cause pain to the individual, commonly around the humeral head in this position. When the compression is almost complete, the practitioner removes their hand and undertakes a final check for skin folds.[1] The breast is compressed to a level that can be tolerated within the required standards: between 9 and 13 daN,[2] and remaining under the maximum level of 20 daN.[3–5]

Essential Image Characteristics

The images should have adequate compression to hold the breast firmly in position with no movement, the breast must be positioned so that the axillary tail is present on the image, with as much of the breast tissue as possible shown.

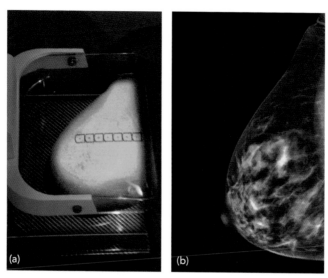

Figure 3.1 (a) Positioning for laterally extended cranio-caudal projection, and (b) corresponding image. (Reproduced from Whitley et al., 2020.)

Additional Considerations

If compression is inadequate, then it may have been too close to the humeral head.

If the breast image shows insufficient axillary tail and axilla, then the nipple was not at the far medial edge of the image receptor before the individual leant back.

If the nipple was not in profile, then the individual did not lean in enough to allow the medial part of the breast to be rotated inwards.

Notes

- Usually, automatic exposure controls are used for standard/routine mammography.
- If imaging implants or medical devices, settings will have to be adjusted.

ADDITIONAL/MODIFIED PROJECTION: CRANIO-CAUDAL – MEDIALLY ROTATED

This is useful for demonstrating lesions in the medial portion of the breast (**Figure 3.2**).

Position of the Individual and Image Receptor

The individual faces the equipment with their sternum about 8 cm (a hands width) from the medial edge of the image receptor. Initially, both breasts are lifted on to the image receptor, which is lowered for this purpose. It is then raised to the correct height, enabling the nipple on the side under examination to be in profile. Consider the techniques used in effective CC positioning (**Figures 3.1, 3.2, and 3.3**).

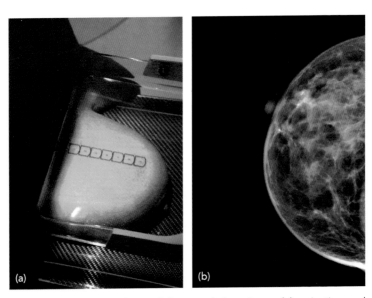

Figure 3.2 (a) Positioning for medially extended cranio-caudal projection, and (b) corresponding image. (Reproduced from Whitley et al., 2020.)

The individual is moved towards the equipment and the breast tissue of the side to be examined moved in and rotated to enable the medial posterior area to be visualised (**Figure 3.2a and b**). The breast is held while the initial compression is applied. Great care must be taken not to cause pain to the individual, commonly around the humeral head and chest wall in this position. When the compression is almost complete, the practitioner removes their hand and undertakes a final check for skin folds.[1] The breast is compressed to a level that can be tolerated within the required standards: between 9 and 13 daN,[2] and remaining under the maximum level of 20 daN.[3-5]

Essential Image Characteristics

The images should have adequate compression to hold the breast firmly in position with no movement. The breast must be positioned to ensure maximum inclusion of the medio-posterior part of the breast.

Additional Considerations

If the inner quadrant is not fully visible, then the individual needs to be encouraged to move further forward into the equipment and the medial part of the breast needs more rotation.

If the nipple was not in profile, then the image receptor was not at the correct height, or the breast was not sufficiently lifted.

Notes

- Usually, automatic exposure controls are used for standard/routine mammography.
- If imaging implants or medical devices, settings will have to be adjusted.

ADDITIONAL/MODIFIED PROJECTION: EXTENDED CRANIO-CAUDAL

The extended CC projection demonstrates the axillary tail and the upper midline portion of the breast tissue.

Position of the Individual and Image Receptor

The image receptor is horizontal and positioned slightly below the infra-mammary angle. The individual stands close to the equipment, with the breast being imaged aligned slightly to the medial side of the midline of the image receptor, their feet and hips towards the image receptor. The individual's breast is lifted and placed on the image receptor while encouraging the individual to lean around 10–15° laterally, extending their arm away from the side of their body. The individual should remain facing the equipment and not rotate obliquely[1] (**Figure 3.3a**).

The breast is held while the initial compression is applied. Great care must be taken not to cause pain to the individual, commonly around the humeral head and chest wall in this position. When the compression is almost complete, the practitioner removes their hand and undertakes a final check for skin folds.[1] The breast is compressed to a level that can be tolerated within the required standards: between 9 and 13 daN,[2] and remaining under the maximum level of 20 daN.[3–5]

Essential Image Characteristics

The images should have adequate compression to hold the breast firmly in position with no movement. The nipple should be in profile and the anterior edge of the pectoral muscle, lateral to the midline of the breast, should be visualised[1] (**Figure 3.3b**).

Additional Considerations

This is a difficult position to achieve and maintain. It is essential that the individual's body remains square to the image receptor and that they do not turn obliquely.

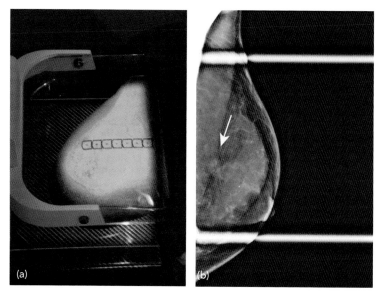

Figure 3.3 (a) Positioning for an extended cranio-caudal projection. (b) Radiograph showing the benefit of extended cranial-caudal projection with magnification showing a distortion (arrow). (Reproduced from Whitley et al., 2020.)

If the nipple is not in profile, then the image receptor was not at the correct height, or the breast was not sufficiently lifted.

Folds in the breast tissue result if the breast was not smoothed out prior to compression application. As skin folds obscure detail, great care must be taken to ensure that they do not occur.

Notes

- Usually, automatic exposure controls are used for standard/routine mammography.
- If imaging implants or medical devices, settings will have to be adjusted.

ADDITIONAL/MODIFIED PROJECTION: LATERAL (MEDIO-LATERAL)

Lateral projections are valuable in localising areas of abnormality, for example micro-calcifications, and in clarification of suspicious lesions. Lateral images are taken at 90° to the CC projection and show the relationship of lesions to the nipple. Both medio-lateral and latero-medial projections can be taken. The medio-lateral is more common; although the axillary area is not demonstrated, overall more of the breast is visualised.[1]

Position of the Individual and Image Receptor

The individual faces the equipment, with the image receptor at the lateral side of the breast, placing their arm behind the image receptor, holding the equipment for stability. The individual leans in from the waist to ensure that the breast tissue closest to the chest wall is visualised; the height of the image receptor is adjusted to the height at which the inferior portion of the breast will be included (**Figure 3.4a**).[1]

The practitioner places their hand on the side of the individual's rib cage and forwards to support the breast tissue of the side being imaged; the palm of the practitioner's hand on the lateral aspect of the individual's breast, thumb on the medial aspect. The individual is moved in gently and the breast extended outwards and upwards against the image receptor, ensuring that the nipple remains in profile. The individual's shoulder of the opposite side is moved backwards so that the compression paddle can be brought into contact with the breast under examination. Firm support of the breast is necessary so the breast tissue at the chest wall margin is not pulled away.[1]

Breast compression is applied gently; when the compression paddle contacts the breast at the chest wall, the individual's other shoulder is brought forwards to ensure that the individual is in a true lateral projection. The breast position is maintained manually. On removing their hand, the practitioner must ensure that the position is maintained when

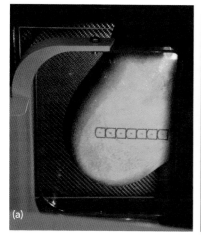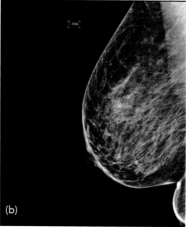

Figure 3.4 (a) Positioning for a medio-lateral projection. (b) Image of a medio-lateral projection. (Reproduced from Whitley et al., 2020.)

final compression is applied. Great care must be taken not to cause discomfort to the individual, commonly near the chest wall. When the compression is almost complete, the practitioner removes their hand and undertakes a final check for skin folds.[1] The breast is compressed to a level that can be tolerated within the required standards: between 9 and 13 daN,[2] and remaining under the maximum level of 20 daN.[3–5]

Essential Image Characteristics

The breast, including its inferior border, should be demonstrated with the same depth of tissue as in the CC projection (**Figure 3.4a and b**).

Additional Considerations

If the nipple of the other breast is demonstrated, then the other breast may need to be held back.[1]

The nipple may not be in profile due to incorrect positioning of the individual:[1]

- if the nipple lies behind the majority of the breast tissue, the individual was too far in front of the image receptor;

- if the nipple lies in front of the majority of the breast tissue, the individual was too far behind the image receptor.

Notes

- Usually, automatic exposure controls are used for standard/routine mammography.
- If imaging implants or medical devices, settings will have to be adjusted.

ADDITIONAL/MODIFIED PROJECTION: LATERAL (LATERO-MEDIAL)

Lateral projections are valuable in localising areas of abnormality, for example, micro-calcifications, and in clarification of suspicious lesions. Lateral images are taken at 90° to the CC projection and show the relationship of lesions to the nipple. This projection is taken for demonstration of medially situated lesions.[1]

Positioning of the Individual and Image Receptor

The individual faces the equipment, with the imaging receptor resting against the sternum, the arm on the side being examined lifted to clear the mammography tube and then rested on to it. The individual's body is rotated inwards slightly to contact the image receptor and the height of the image receptor is adjusted to the height at which the lower border of the breast will be included (**Figure 3.5a**).

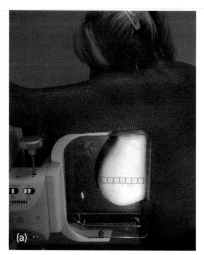
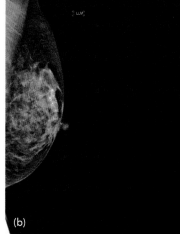

Figure 3.5 (a) Positioning for a latero-medial projection. (b) Image of a latero-medial projection. (Reproduced from Whitley et al., 2020.)

55

The individual's breast is gently guided across and upwards, ensuring that their nipple remains in profile. Breast compression is applied gently and when the compression paddle contacts the breast, on removing their hand, the practitioner must ensure that the individual's position is maintained as final compression is applied. Great care must be taken not to cause pain to the individual. When the compression is almost complete, the practitioner removes their hand and undertakes a final check for skin folds.[1] The breast is compressed to a level that can be tolerated within the required standards: between 9 and 13 daN,[2] and remaining under the maximum level of 20 daN.[3–5]

Essential Image Characteristics

The breast is demonstrated fully, including its inferior border, with the same depth of tissue as in the CC projection (**Figure 3.5b**).

Additional Considerations

If the nipple was not in profile, then the individual's arm was pulled over too much, thus rotating the body into an oblique position and causing the nipple to lie under the majority of the breast tissue.[1]

Folds in the breast tissue result if the breast was not smoothed out prior to compression application. As skin folds obscure detail, great care must be taken to ensure that they do not occur.[1]

Notes

- Usually, automatic exposure controls are used for standard/routine mammography.
- If imaging implants or medical devices, settings will have to be adjusted.

ADDITIONAL/MODIFIED PROJECTION: AXILLARY TAIL

This projection is valuable in individuals where lymph gland involvement of a breast carcinoma is suspected or there is accessory breast tissue, as it demonstrates tissue high into the axilla.[1]

Positioning of the Individual and Image Receptor

The mammography unit is initially set at an angle of around 45°. The individual faces the equipment with their feet turned to an angle of approximately 15° towards the midline. Raising the arm under the side of examination, it is often helpful at this stage to ask the individual to rest their palm on their head. Remaining close to the mammography equipment, the individual is leant forwards so that the corner of the image receptor rests in the axilla.

The practitioner should then adjust the individual's arm so that their humeral head rests across the top of the image receptor and the corner of the image receptor lies within the axilla. The individual is then encouraged to lean against the image receptor, their breast tissue held forward by the practitioner to ensure an even thickness and to improve the compression of the axillary region. Breast compression is applied gently, and when the compression paddle contacts the breast, on removing their hand, the practitioner must ensure that the individual's position is maintained as final compression is applied (**Figure 3.6a**). Great care must be taken not to cause pain to the individual.

Essential Image Characteristics

The axillary region must be demonstrated (**Figure 3.6b**).

Additional Considerations

Inadequate compression can occur, this is often due to the humeral head or the clavicle being caught by the compression paddle due to poor positioning.[1]

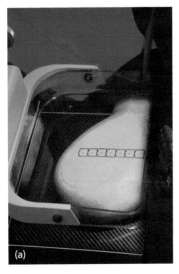 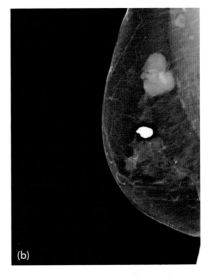

Figure 3.6 (a) Positioning for an axillary tail projection. (b) Image of an axillary tail projection. (Reproduced from Whitley et al., 2020.)

Folds in the breast tissue result if the breast was not smoothed out prior to compression application. As skin folds obscure detail, great care must be taken to ensure that they do not occur.[1]

Notes

- Usually, automatic exposure controls are used for standard/routine mammography.
- If imaging implants or medical devices, settings will have to be adjusted.

ADDITIONAL/MODIFIED PROJECTION: LOCALISED COMPRESSION/PADDLE

Localised compression/paddle projections can provide extra information in a suspicious area, for example they can demonstrate whether the borders of a lesion are defined clearly or indistinctly. The paddle projections required are usually selected with the aim of repeating those projections that initially demonstrated the possible lesion. For accurate localisation of the region of interest, the original mammogram must be compared. It is essential that the practitioner measures and records the depth of the lesion from the nipple back towards the chest wall, the distance of the lesion from the nipple (above, below, medial, or lateral), and the distance from the skin surface to the lesion.[1]

Positioning of the Individual and Image Receptor

The individual is positioned as for the original projection and the recorded coordinates used to position the individual until the affected breast tissue lies over the automatic exposure control and the compression paddle is centred over it.

Allowances must be made for the coordinates being recorded from a fully compressed breast; sufficient compression is applied to hold the breast in place and the coordinates rechecked. Provided that the region of interest is centred under the paddle, the centring point is marked on the skin surface and compression applied. If the area of interest was not under the paddle on checking, then the individual's position is adjusted before proceeding. The compression will feel quite uncomfortable to the individual as a small area of the breast is being compressed; with the force being applied to only a small area, the pressure applied will be high. This should be explained to the individual and they should be reassured that this will only be for a short time.

Essential Image Characteristics

The localised area to be imaged should be clearly demonstrated in the centre of the compressed area (as demonstrated in **Figure 3.7a, b**).

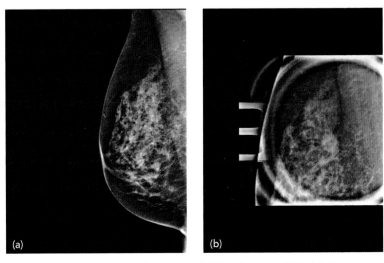

Figure 3.7 (a) Mammogram showing an ill-defined region. (b) Paddle image using paddle compression to show the effect of compression. (Reproduced from Whitley et al., 2020.)

Additional Considerations

Folds in the breast tissue result if the breast was not smoothed out prior to compression application. As skin folds obscure detail, great care must be taken to ensure that they do not occur.[1]

If the region of interest is not centred under the paddle, it is often better to go back to the original mammography image and re-measure the coordinates and then re-measure on the individual.

Notes

- If imaging implants or medical devices, settings will have to be adjusted.

ADDITIONAL/MODIFIED PROJECTION: MAGNIFIED

Projections of the breast using a magnification technique are sometimes employed to provide enhanced visualisation of the breast architecture and detail, thus promoting better diagnosis. Although there is a reduction in the need for magnification projections, conventional magnification mammography frequently remains the technique of choice for detail and clarity of shape and margins, especially for micro-calcifications.[1]

Positioning of the Individual and Image Receptor

As with standard paddle projections, the recording of the coordinates of the lesion from the original images and the positioning technique is essential to accurately centre the lesion under the paddle. For magnified projections, the use of a fine focus will lengthen the exposure time greatly, and the projections should be taken on arrested respiration.

Essential Image Characteristics

The localised area to be imaged should be clearly demonstrated in the centre of the compressed area (as demonstrated in **Figure 3.8**).

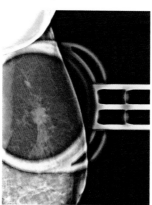

Figure 3.8 Mammogram demonstrating paddle magnification. (Reproduced from Whitley et al., 2020.)

Additional Considerations

Magnified projections are undertaken in the CC and medio-lateral projections. A fine focus of 0.1 mm^2 is essential, and a magnification factor of 2 is commonly used. Magnification factors are typically 1.5, 1.8, or 2.0.

Folds in the breast tissue result if the breast was not smoothed out prior to compression application. As skin folds obscure detail, great care must be taken to ensure that they do not occur.[1]

If the region of interest is not centred under the paddle, it is often better to go back to the original mammography image and re-measure the coordinates and then re-measure on the individual.

Notes

■ If imaging implants or medical devices, settings will have to be adjusted.

STEREOTACTIC PROCEDURES

Due to improvements in the technical quality of mammography, an increasing number of clinically impalpable breast lesions are being detected. These, like palpable lesions, require further radiological investigation to establish a diagnosis. Commonly, further mammographic projections and ultrasound examinations are undertaken to confirm the presence of the suspected abnormality and to assess its clinical importance. Any impalpable lesion that cannot be stated definitively to be benign after such procedures must have a tissue diagnosis.[1] This is achieved by:

- image-guided fine needle aspiration (FNA) cytology; and/or
- image-guided core biopsy (CB) wherever possible (**Figure 3.9**).

Open surgical biopsy is thus avoided. While FNA or CB can be undertaken freehand in palpable lesions, impalpable lesions produce unique problems. FNA has been replaced by CB in many centres using a wide gauge (14) core cut or 11 gauge mammotome device for diagnosis.

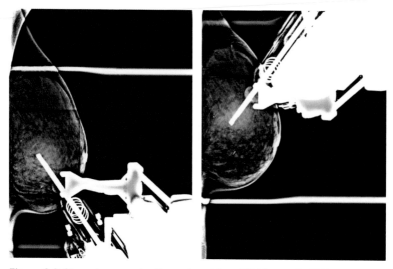

Figure 3.9 Stereo image pair. (Reproduced from Whitley et al., 2020.)

Ultrasound-guided biopsy is preferable for impalpable lesions, as it is quick to perform, very accurate, and associated with minimal discomfort and morbidity. It is the guidance technique of choice for biopsy if the lesion is visualised clearly on ultrasound. X-ray-guided FNA or CB is essential if there is any doubt that what is seen on ultrasound is the same lesion as that visualised on the mammograms, and when the lesion is not demonstrated on ultrasound.[1]

The most accurate way of performing X-ray-guided FNA or CB is using stereotactic equipment. Accuracy is essential to ensure the relevant area is sampled, as the definitive treatment is based on the outcome of the cytological/histological sample. There are two main types of stereotactic equipment: a purpose-built table on which the individual lies prone, and an accessory that is fitted to conventional mammographic equipment.[1]

Positioning of the Individual and Image Receptor

Agreement on positioning is agreed with the practitioner/radiologist undertaking the procedure. The individual is seated and positioned – it is imperative at this stage that they are comfortable as this position must be maintained; ensure positioning aids and pillows are available. Compression is then applied using the compression paddle with the integral window.

An outline of the compression plate window is drawn on to the individual's skin to ensure any breast movement during the procedure is evident. The mammography tube movements necessary to produce the stereo images are performed (typically swung 20° to each side of the midline). The images are checked with the practitioner/radiologist performing the procedure, ensuring that the lesion is shown clearly and that it is not too close to the edge of the compression plate window. The coordinates of the lesion will be calculated by the equipment from the stereo images. A local anaesthetic injection to the skin over the biopsy area is given by the practitioner/radiologist performing the procedure.[1]

The coordinates are sent to the mammography machine and the practitioner/radiologist performing the procedure places the needle in the breast. A check image is essential after the needle has been placed to confirm needle location (**Figure 3.9**).[1] The aspiration or CB sample is taken and the procedure may be repeated with several passes to gain multiple samples. A marker clip can then be deployed for future reference prior to localisation (**Figure 3.10**).[1]

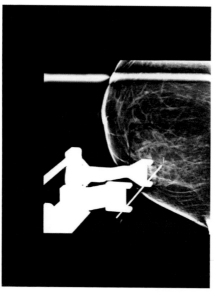

Figure 3.10 Image demonstrating marker clip. (Reproduced from Whitley et al., 2020.)

Essential Image Characteristics

Modern equipment has a digital system for biopsy and spot imaging. Historic film processing has been replaced with digital image acquisition and reconstruction, which is completed swiftly and accurately.

Additional Considerations

Those undergoing this procedure will be anxious; a good rapport between the individual and the practitioner is essential. A thorough explanation of the procedure before it commences and at each step along the way is important as this will relax and reassure the individual.

Notes

- The set-up for stereotactic preoperative wire or marker localisation procedures is similar to that described for stereotactic FNA or CB.
- The marker wire that is used instead of the fine needle or the biopsy gun will depend on the preferences of the surgeon performing the biopsy or excision.
- The purpose of this localisation is for a marker wire to be placed accurately in the breast lesion so that the surgeon can perform a diagnostic biopsy of the lesion.
- It is essential that the marker wire tip lies within the lesion, so that accurate assessment is made of the depth of the abnormality in the compressed breast.
- The position of the wire in relation to the abnormality in the breast must therefore be checked mammographically after marker insertion (**Figure 3.11**).

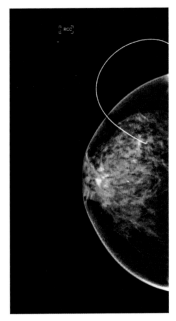

Figure 3.11 Image demonstrating localisation marker wire. (Reproduced from Whitley et al., 2020.)

SPECIMEN TISSUE IMAGING

Both CB and specimen breast radiography, involving a magnification technique, play an important role in the diagnosis, management, and treatment of breast cancer. Breast tissue cores are examined radiographically to determine the presence of a breast lesion that may contain or be solely composed of calcifications.[1]

Position of a Specimen on the Image Receptor

Following a CB, the excised tissue cores are laid out on a fibre-free sheet or in a dedicated specimen holder kept moist with isotonic saline to prevent desiccation (**Figure 3.12**). Imaging may be performed on the mammography table using the magnification facility or within a specimen radiography cabinet. Once adequate images have been obtained, the tissue cores must be transferred to a fixative, usually formalin, and transported to the laboratory immediately for processing for subsequent histology.[1]

Following excision of a breast abnormality in theatre, the breast tissue specimen is sent for radiographic examination (**Figure 3.13**) while

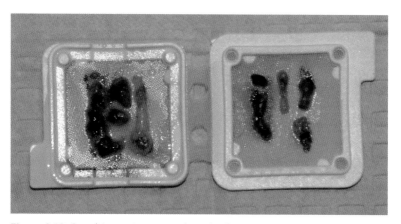

Figure 3.12 Core biopsy tissue sample within biopsy container. (Reproduced from Whitley et al., 2020.)

the patient is still under anaesthetic; the procedure is therefore carried out as quickly and as efficiently as possible. Current guidelines state that to ensure adequate surgical excision of an invasive cancer treated by breast conservation surgery, all patients should have their tumours removed with no evidence of disease at the microscopic radial margins and fulfilling the requirements of local guidelines. If, after multidisciplinary meeting discussion, the margin of excision is deemed to be inadequate, then further surgery to obtain clear margins should be recommended.[1]

It is imperative that the image and any corresponding biopsy sample are correctly labelled with the patient identification and laterality of tissue sample as per guidelines prior to sending to histopathology.

Additional Considerations

Immediate specimen radiography of surgical specimens from impalpable lesions will be assessed to confirm that they include the radiological abnormality.[6] Following excision of the breast abnormality, the breast tissue specimen is sent for radiographic examination (**Figure 3.13**) while the patient is still under anaesthetic, thus, the procedure is carried out as quickly and as efficiently as possible.

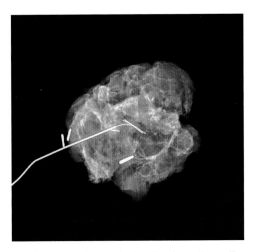

Figure 3.13 Image demonstrating a wire localised specimen. (Reproduced from Whitley et al., 2020.)

68

Current guidelines state that to ensure adequate surgical excision of an invasive cancer treated by breast conservation surgery, all patients should have their tumours removed with no evidence of disease at the microscopic radial margins and fulfilling the requirements of local guidelines. If, after multidisciplinary meeting discussion, the margin of excision is deemed to be inadequate, then further surgery to obtain clear margins should be recommended.

National Institute for Health and Care Excellence (NICE) guidelines further state that a minimum of 2 mm radial margin of excision is recommended with pathological examination to National Health Service Breast Screening Programme (NHSBSP) reporting standards. Re-excision should be considered if the margin is less than 2 mm, following discussion of the risks and benefits with the patient.[7]

REFERENCES

1. Whitley, S.A., Dodgeon, J., Meadows, A., Cullingworth, J., Holmes, K., Jackson, M., Hoadley, G. and Kulshrestha, R. *Clark's Procedures in Diagnostic Imaging: A System-Based Approach.* CRC Press, 2020.

2. Hogg, P., Taylor, M., Szczepura, K., Mercer, C., and Denton, E. Pressure and breast thickness in mammography—an exploratory calibration study. *The British Journal of Radiology* 2013;86(1021):20120222. https://www.birpublications.org/doi/10.1259/bjr.20120222.

3. European Commission Initiative on Breast Cancer. European guidelines on breast cancer screening and diagnosis. 2021. Available at: https://healthcare-quality.jrc.ec.europa.eu/ecibc/european-breast-cancer-guidelines.

4. Public Health England. Breast screening: guidance for breast screening mammographers. 2020. Available at: https://www.gov.uk/government/publications/breast-screening-quality-assurance-for-mammography-and-radiography.

5. Mercer, C., Hogg, P., and Kelly, J. *Digital Mammography: A Holistic Approach.* 2nd edition. UK: Springer, 2022.

6. Public Health England. Breast Screening; quality assurance guidelines for breast pathology services. 2020. Available at: https://www.gov.uk/government/publications/breast-screening-quality-assurance-guidelines-for-breast-pathology-services.

7. National Institute for Health and Care Excellence. NICE guideline 101. Early and locally advanced breast cancer, diagnosis and treatment. 2018. Available at: https://www.nice.org.uk/guidance/ng101.

SECTION 4

USEFUL INFORMATION FOR MAMMOGRAPHIC PRACTICE

MEDICAL TERMINOLOGY[1]

Abscess
A closed pocket containing pus (a creamy, thick, pale yellow or yellow-green fluid that comes from dead tissue; commonly caused by a bacterial infection).

Adenocarcinoma
Cancer arising in gland-forming tissue. Breast cancer is a type of adenocarcinoma.

Adenoma
A non-cancerous tumour made up of glandular tissue (such as breast, lung, thyroid, colon, pancreas).

Adenopathy
Enlargement of the lymph nodes.

Adhesion
Cell attachment to neighbouring structures. One of the necessary steps to a cancer growing.

Adjuvant
Something that enhances the effectiveness of medical treatment, i.e., chemotherapy, radiation, tamoxifen.

Adjuvant chemotherapy
Anticancer drugs used in combination with surgery and/or radiation as an initial treatment before there is detectable spread, to prevent or delay recurrence.

Adjuvant therapy
1. The use of an antigen that increases the specific immune response to antigens.
2. Therapy given following surgery to help prevent a cancer's recurrence or to destroy cancer cells that have metastasised. Chemotherapy, radiation, and hormonal therapies are examples.

Allergic reaction to chemotherapy
Chemotherapy can cause an allergic reaction in some patients. This is not always predictable and usually occurs within the first 15–30 minutes of drug administration. There are usually no long-term effects from the complication; however, future administration of the same drug may not be possible.

Areola
Circular pigmented area around the nipple that contains sweat glands and sebaceous glands.

Atypia
A condition of being irregular or non-standard, e.g. abnormality in a cell.

Axilla
The hollow of the armpit – region between the arm and the thoracic wall.

Benign
Not cancerous.

Benign breast disease
Most breast complaints are benign in nature. Despite this, most women with breast complaints 'assume the worst' when a new problem is discovered.

Bilateral
Involving both sides, such as both breasts.

Biomarkers
Tests to identify characteristics of tumour cells.

Biopsy
Removal of tissue. This term does not indicate how much tissue will be removed, i.e., core biopsy, excision biopsy, fine needle biopsy, stereotactic biopsy, surgical biopsy, punch biopsy, wire localisation biopsy.

Blood count
The number of red blood cells, white blood cells, and platelets in a sample of blood.

Calcifications
Calcium deposits in non-bony tissue. Breast calcifications are sometimes found by mammography.

Calcium
A chemical element that is a major component of bone. Calcium does not in itself prevent osteoporosis but it is recommended for prevention, and in treatment, of osteoporosis.

Cancer
A multistep genetic disease resulting from specific alterations in the function of one or more genes, disrupting the control of cellular growth and differentiation.

Carcinogen
Substance or physical agent (such as ionising radiation) that can cause cancer.

Carcinoma
Cancer arising in the skin, glands, and lining of internal organs. Most cancers are carcinomas.

Carcinoma in situ
Cancer that is confined to the cells where it began and has not spread into surrounding tissue.

DCIS
Ductal carcinoma in situ – cancer confined to within the ductal system of the breast.

Differentiated
Clearly defined. Differentiated tumour cells are similar in appearance to normal cells.

Disease-free survival
Time the patient survives without any detectable cancer after initial treatment.

Dissection
Removal of specific tissue (breast lump), leaving surrounding tissues in place.

DNA
1. Deoxyribonucleic acid – a molecule that carries genetic information.
2. Did not attend, if talking about clients not attending screening invitations.

Effusion
A collection of fluid in a body cavity, usually between two adjoining tissues. For example, a pleural effusion is the collection of fluid between two layers of the pleura (the lung's covering).

Encapsulated
Confined to a specific area; the tumour remains in a compact form.

Endocrine therapy
Hormone-altering drugs used to treat breast cancer. Endocrine therapy is also referred to as hormone therapy or hormone treatment.

Enzyme
A protein molecule that accelerates chemical reactions in cells or organisms.

Erythema
Redness of the skin.

Excise
To cut or remove surgically.

Familial cancer
A form of cancer that occurs in various members of the same family at a significantly higher rate than can be expected to occur by chance.

Family history
Clinical history where family members are identified as having breast disease.

Fascia
A fibrous membrane covering, supporting, and separating muscles and various organs of the body, which attaches the breasts and other body structures to underlying muscles.

Fat necrosis
A section of dead fat usually resulting from some kind of trauma or surgery that can appear as a thickened area or lump(s).

Fibroadenoma

A common non-malignant lump. This is a smooth, hard, and round lump that feels the way most people think a cyst should feel. It moves around easily within the breast tissue and is often found near the nipple. Fibroadenomas are benign and are most common in young women.

Fibrocystic disease

Much misused term for any benign condition of the breast.

Fine needle biopsy or aspiration (FNB or FNA)

In a fine needle biopsy of a lump, the radiologist/surgeon anaesthetises the breast with a small amount of lignocaine and then uses a needle and syringe to collect a few cells. When examined, this often shows whether something is benign or cancerous.

Flap

A portion of tissue with its own blood supply moved from one part of the body to another. Flaps of muscle, fat, and skin are often used in reconstructive breast surgery to provide additional tissue for the reconstructed breast. Common donor sites are abdomen, back, and buttocks.

Genetic risk factors

Three types of genetic factors:
1. Sporadic: 70% of breast cancer patients who have no family history.
2. Genetic: one dominant cancer gene and passed on to every generation.
3. Polygenic: occurs when there is family history that is not directly passed on.

Gluteal musculocutaneous free flap

One of the techniques for breast reconstruction which uses the patient's own tissues rather than an implant.

Grade

A measure of how normal or abnormal cancer cells look under a microscope. This is also called the histological grade and is done by the pathologist when examining the tumour biopsy. Breast cancer tumours are graded on a scale of 1 to 3. Grade 1 tumours appear most like normal tissue (well-differentiated). Grade 3 tumours appear very abnormal (poorly differentiated). May predict aggressiveness.

HER2, HER2/neu
The name for a growth factor receptor.

Heterogeneous
Composed of many different elements. In relation to breast cancer, heterogeneous refers to the fact that there are many different types of breast cancer cells within one tumour.

Hormone
Chemical substance produced by glands in the body, which enters the bloodstream and causes effects in other tissues.

Hormone receptor test
A test to measure the amount of certain proteins, called hormone receptors, in breast cancer tissue. Hormones can attach to these proteins. A high level of hormone receptors means hormones probably help the cancer to grow.

Hormone replacement therapy (HRT)
As a woman reaches menopause (typically around 50), her body produces less of the female hormone oestrogen. HRT is designed to replace female hormones that the ovaries produce before menopause.

Immune system
Complex system by which the body can protect itself from foreign invaders.

Immunodeficiency
A lowering of the body's ability to fight off infection and disease.

Immunotherapy
Genetically re-engineered genes are used to boost the immune system. This is designed to act only on the cancer cells, so there is no adverse effect on normal cells, thus there are no adverse side effects.

Implant
A silicone gel-filled or saline-filled sac inserted under the chest muscle to restore breast shape.

Infiltrating cancer
Cancer that has grown through the basement membrane at its site of origin into neighbouring tissue. Infiltrating does not imply that the

cancer has already spread outside the breast. Infiltrating has the same meaning as invasive.

Inflammatory breast cancer

A warm swollen breast that does not change through the menstrual cycle or respond to antibiotics. Skin which is red or appears dimpled like an orange – 'peau d'orange'.

Infraclavicular nodes

Lymph nodes lying below the collarbone.

In situ

'In the site of'. For cancer, in situ refers to tumours that have not grown beyond their site of origin and thus not invaded neighbouring tissue.

Invasive ductal carcinoma (IDC)

Begins in the milk ducts of the breast and penetrates the wall of the duct, invading the fatty tissue of the breast and possibly other regions of the body. It is the most common type of breast cancer, accounting for 80% of breast cancer diagnoses.

Invasive lobular carcinoma (ILC)

Begins in the milk glands (lobules) of the breast, but often spreads to other regions of the body. It accounts for 10–15% of breast cancers.

Latissimus flap

Flap of skin and muscle taken from the back and used for reconstruction after mastectomy or partial mastectomy.

Leukopenia

Leukocytes are white blood cells. A decrease in the number of white blood cells is called leukopenia. White blood cells fight bacteria that enter the body and are the body's main defence against infection. White blood cells are made inside the bones in the soft, spongy material called bone marrow. When white blood cells are decreased because of chemotherapy and radiotherapy, the risk of infection increases.

Lobular carcinoma

A type of breast cancer that begins in the milk-producing glands (lobules) of the breast. An invasive tumour and normally presents as a diffuse swelling rather than a discrete lump; in many cases there are tumours in both breasts. It is somewhat difficult to detect on mammography in comparison to ductal cancers due to indiscrete borders. However, compared to ductal carcinoma, lobular carcinoma is associated with a better prognosis.

Lobular carcinoma in situ (LCIS)
Considered pre-cancer, this 'marker' is located in the deeper areas where milk production starts. Believed to carry a small risk (20%) over a lifetime, of developing into invasive cancer.

Lobules
Parts of the breast capable of making milk. Look like a 'bunch of grapes'.

Local recurrence
Redevelopment of a tumour at a site where it had initially been removed.

Lumpectomy
Surgery to remove a lump with a small rim of normal tissue around it.

Lymph
The almost colourless fluid that travels through the lymphatic system and carries cells that helps to fight infection and disease.

Lymph node dissection
When the surgeon removes several lymph nodes during either a mastectomy or lumpectomy so that the pathologist can dissect the node into thin slices, which are then stained and examined to look for cancerous cells.

Lymph nodes
Glands found throughout the body that help defend against foreign invaders such as bacteria. Lymph nodes can be a location of cancer spread.

Lymphatic vessels
Vessels that carry lymph (tissue fluid) to and from lymph nodes.

Lymphocytes
White blood cells made in lymphatic tissue and distributed throughout the body by way of the lymphatic fluid and blood.

Lymphoedema

'Milk arm'. This swelling of the arm can follow surgery to the lymph nodes under the arm. It can be temporary or permanent and occur immediately or any time later.

Macro-calcifications

Larger, coarse calcium deposits that are often related to benign (non-cancerous) growths such as fibroadenomas or degenerative changes in the breasts, such as ageing of the breast arteries, old injuries, or inflammation. Macro-calcifications are usually associated with benign (non-cancerous) conditions and may not require a biopsy.

Magnetic resonance imaging (MRI)

A technique used to provide image information of the brain, soft tissues, large blood vessels, and/or the heart. It involves the use of a magnetic field and electrical coil to transmit radio waves throughout the body.

Malignant

Cancerous.

Mammogram – stereotactic

Many percutaneous biopsy procedures are performed with the help of some form of image guidance, which typically includes ultrasound and computed tomography (CT). Many breast biopsies are performed under the guidance of stereotactic mammography.

Mammography

An X-ray of the breast. Digital (computerised) mammography is similar to analogue mammography in that X-rays are used to produce detailed images of the breast.

Margins

An area next to a tumour. It is important to have 'clean margins' after a lumpectomy, i.e., an amount of cancer-free tissue must be removed with the tumour.

Mastalgia

Pain in the breast.

Mastectomy

Surgical removal of the breast. Includes modified radical mastectomy, radical mastectomy, partial mastectomy, wide local excision mastectomy, and lumpectomy.

Mastectomy, modified radical

The most common mastectomy procedure. It involves the removal of the breast and the lymph nodes in the armpit.

Mastectomy, radical

This procedure is more rarely done. It involves the removal of the breast, muscle of the chest wall, and enough skin to require a skin graft.

Necrosis

Death of, or in, tissue.

Neoadjuvant chemotherapy

Chemotherapy given before breast cancer surgery. Also called 'primary chemotherapy' or 'induction chemotherapy'. In some cases of breast cancer, the large size of the cancer or the extent of involvement in the breast, chest wall, or axilla are such that surgery cannot be performed at the time of diagnosis. By giving three to four treatments of chemotherapy first, the cancer may shrink so that surgery can be performed.

Neoplasm

A new and abnormal formation of tissue, such as a tumour or growth. It serves no useful purpose but grows at the expense of the healthy organism.

Nipple

The conical projection in the centre of the breast, containing the outlets of the milk ducts.

Nipple discharge

Nipple discharge is the third most common breast complaint for which women seek medical attention, after lumps and breast pain.

Non-invasive

Self-contained, not growing into or destroying healthy tissue.

Nuclear grade
In a pathologist report meaning the number of cells dividing and the manner in which they divide. Aggressive cancer tends to have a lot of cells dividing, less aggressive cancers tend to have fewer. Usually graded on a scale of 1 to 3 or 1 to 4, with higher numbers indicating worst prognosis.

Nuclear medicine breast imaging
Involves the injection into the body of very tiny amounts of a radioactive substance linked with a second substance that collects in the targeted organ.

Oestrogen receptor (ER)
Significant levels of ERs have been observed in a large percentage of breast cancers. The receptor can be (+) positive or (–) negative. Most (+) receptor tumours respond better to treatment, so receptor status is used as a prognostic marker for recurrence.

Oncogene
Tumour genes present in the body. These can be activated by carcinogens and cause cells to grow uncontrollably.

Oncology/oncologist
Study of cancer.

Oophorectomy
Surgical removal of ovaries.

Osteopathy
A system of medical therapy based on the belief that the body is capable of making its own remedies against disease when its parts are in a normal structural relationship and have favourable environmental conditions and adequate nutrition.

Osteoporosis
Softening of the bones that occurs with age in some people.

Ovarian ablation
Ovarian ablation or castration refers to a medical procedure to remove or inactivate the ovaries and prevent their ability to produce oestrogen. Ovarian ablation can be accomplished by surgery (called oophorectomy), radiation therapy, or by the administration of special

hormone-altering medications. This procedure is a hormone therapy treatment for pre-menopausal women with breast cancer whose cancers are oestrogen receptor positive or of unknown status.

Paget's disease of the breast
A form of breast cancer that shows up in the nipple as an itchiness and scaling that does not get better, and is often mistaken for eczema of the nipple. It is almost never found in both breasts (bilateral).

Pain (breast)
Breast pain (mastalgia) is the most common breast-related complaint among women.

Palliative care
Refers to any treatment with the goal of symptom relief and comfort to improve quality of life, rather than to cure.

Palpable
Can be felt.

Papillary carcinoma
Cancer that has cells that stick out in little papules, or finger-like projections.

Pathological fracture
Fracture of a bone caused by something being wrong with the bone itself, not by an outside blunt trauma. Differing from osteoporosis in that it does not affect all bones.

Pathologist
A physician who specialises in the diagnosis and classification of diseases by using laboratory tests to determine the origin of the disease and whether or not it is invasive (has invaded nearby tissues in the breast) and assign a grade to the breast tumour to identify the type of tumour present and help recommend a treatment plan for an optimal outcome.

Pathology report
A report of the analysis of cells and tissues to determine what disease conditions may be present. The report will state whether the tissue is cancerous, pre-cancerous, or benign. If cancerous, it will give information to estimate how aggressive the tumour is, whether it has passed

through the basement membrane and begun to invade adjacent tissue, and whether cancer is at or close to the edges of the block tissue that was removed.

Peau d'orange
Dimpling of the breast skin caused by swelling (oedema) where the tumour is. The ligaments that hold the breast tissue to the skin get pulled in, and this gives the skin the dimpled 'orange peel' appearance.

Pectoralis major
Muscle that lies under the breast.

Quadrantectomy
Removal of a quarter of the breast; a form of lumpectomy.

Radiation pneumonitis
If the lung or parts of the lung are included in the radiation treatment field, as is the case with breast cancer, the radiation can cause inflammation or irritation of the lung tissue, which is called 'radiation pneumonitis'. This potential complication usually occurs about six months or longer after the completion of radiation therapy.

Radiation skin reactions
Skin changes can occur with external beam radiation therapy. Radiation therapy may irritate the skin in the treatment area causing redness, warmth, swelling, dry or moist peeling, itching, irritation of the hair pores in the treatment area, and ulceration. Hair loss around the nipple and the axilla may also occur. These changes may cause some temporary mild discomfort but will resolve once treatment is completed and the skin has time to heal.

Radiation soft tissue fibrosis
Radiation therapy can cause changes in the soft tissue of the breast and/or chest wall resulting in scarring of the tissue. The skin and tissue underneath may feel thickened, firm, and tight, and spidery purple-red blood vessels may develop in the area. These tissue changes may result in the breast becoming smaller. The skin in this area will be more sensitive and should be protected from sun exposure and injury.

Radiation therapy
A local therapy for breast cancer. Typically, radiation is one component of primary therapy for breast cancer that usually follows surgical procedures such as lumpectomy or mastectomy, and may be accompanied by chemotherapy. In some instances where surgery is not possible or a patient refuses surgery, radiation is used to treat the primary tumour itself. Usually consisting of high-voltage X-rays, radiation kills dividing cells by inducing DNA damage.

Receptor
In pharmacology, a cell component that joins with a drug, hormone, or chemical mediator to alter the function of the cell.

Reconstruction
Creation of artificial breast after mastectomy by a plastic surgeon.

Reconstructive/plastic surgeon
If the breast is removed (mastectomy) as part of treatment, a plastic surgeon may perform breast reconstruction in many instances.

Saline implants
Similar to silicone implants, except that saline (salt water), not silicone gel, is in the silicone shell. Saline is no less likely to leak than silicone, but when it does, it becomes absorbed by the body fairly quickly causing no medical problems.

Sarcoma
A malignant tumour arising in the connective tissue.

Screening
Use of a test to check for disease when there are no signs of symptoms.

Secondary malignancy (cancer)
Radiation therapy and chemotherapy can cause changes in the structure and DNA of normal cells. Sometimes these changes cannot be repaired, and over time, these cells undergo more changes and eventually transform into a malignant or cancerous cell and tumour. These secondary cancers, caused by the initial cancer treatment, usually occur five or six years after therapy is completed. However, some may be as early as several years or as long as 10 or 12 years.

Segmentectomy
Removal of a segment of breast tissue; usually the same as a lumpectomy.

Self-examination
Regular 'self' breast checks/examinations to know 'what is normal' for the individual and therefore detect any changes at an earlier stage.

Sentinel lymph node surgery
Removal of the sentinel or guard node.

Sentinel node biopsy (mapping)
Mapping the regional lymphatics (lymph nodes) with a blue dye to predict presence or absence of regional nodal metastases in patients with breast cancer. This technique involves injecting dye near a tumour and within a few hours removing the tumour, and the sentinel node(s) most likely to contain metastasis. Advantages of this procedure over complete axillary dissection include faster recovery and no nerve damage to the arm. Sentinel lymph node mapping has been shown to eliminate the risk of lymphoedema.

Seroma
A sac or cyst filled with blood serum. Seromas often occur in the potential space where the skin flaps of a mastectomy have not yet adhered to the chest wall. Drains are often left in place to remove the fluid so that the skin flap can stick to the chest wall.

Silicone
Synthetic material used in breast implants because of its flexibility, resilience, and durability.

Skin flap necrosis
The skin over the incision site and surgical area may not get enough blood supply after surgery. When this happens, the 'skin flap' in this area may begin to develop areas where the tissue dies and turns dusky or dark.

Tamoxifen
Oestrogen blocker used in treating breast cancer.

Tamoxifen response
The time (in months to years) between the completion of tamoxifen therapy and the point at which the cancer returned. This information

is important for the doctor in determining whether tamoxifen can be used again to treat a cancer recurrence.

Thermography

A test to measure and display heat patterns of tissues near the surface of the breast. Abnormal tissue generally is warmer than healthy tissue. This technique is under study; its value in detecting breast cancer has not been proven.

Tissue expander

A variation on a breast implant used in reconstruction. An empty sack is placed behind the muscle, everything is sewn closed and gradually, over three to six months, saline solution is injected through a tube. The temporary implant is then removed and replaced with a permanent saline implant or silicone implant.

Toxicity

Harmful side effects, poisonous.

Ultrasound

Breast ultrasound is frequently used to evaluate breast abnormalities. It uses sound waves and their echoes to form images.

WBC (white blood cell) count

A blood test to measure the number of white blood cells in the blood. White blood cells are part of the immune system that are important in resistance to infections.

White blood cells

Blood cells that fight infection and are made in the bone marrow, along with red blood cells and platelets. When there are not enough white blood cells due to disease or the effects of cancer treatment such as chemotherapy or radiation therapy, there is an increased risk of developing an infection.

Wire localisation biopsy

Used when a lesion is not palpable (cannot be felt). A thin wire is inserted through a needle, directed by use of imaging, to direct the surgeon to the lesion.

REFERENCE

1. Whitley, S.A., Dodgeon, J., Meadows, A., Cullingworth, J., Holmes, K., Jackson, M., Hoadley, G., and Kulshrestha, R. *Clark's Procedures in Diagnostic Imaging: A System-Based Approach*. CRC Press, 2020.

INDEX